PRIMAL PATTERN® EATING

PRIMAL PATTERN® EATING

Ditch the diet B.S. and learn how to eat the way you were born to

PAUL CHEK

Primal Pattern® Eating

Cover design: Ali Arthington, Thoughtful Creative Limited
Book design: Adina Cucicov
Editors: Penthea Crozier & Phil Delaire

C.H.E.K Institute
San Diego, CA, USA
+1.760.477.2620
info@chekinstitute.com
www.chekinstitute.com
Printed in the USA

Tradepaper ISBN: 978-1-58387-019-8
Digital pdf ISBN: 978-1-58387-020-4
epub ISBN: 978-1-58387-021-1
Chek, Paul W.

Warning—Disclaimer
The workouts and other health-related activities described in this book was developed by the author and are to be used as an adjunct to improved strengthening, conditioning, health and fitness regimens. These programs may not be appropriate for everyone. All individuals, especially those who suffer from any disease or are recovering from any injury, should consult their physicians regarding the advisability of undertaking any of the activities suggested in these programs. The author has been painstaking in his research. However, he is neither responsible nor liable for any harm or injury resulting from this program or the use of the exercises or exercise devices described herein.

TABLE OF CONTENTS

CHAPTER 1

IS THERE A PERFECT DIET FOR EVERYONE?

"Tell me what you eat, and I will tell you what you are."

~ Anthelme Brillat-Savarin, The Physiology of Taste, 1825

In a world saturated with diet books and wellness options, each promising a one-size-fits-all solution, it's tempting to believe that the secret to health lies in a singular method. But can any one diet truly serve all people equally?

The truth is that human beings are exquisitely unique, biologically, emotionally, and mentally. Our bodies operate within vastly different environments, and our individual needs are shaped by a complex interplay of genetics, lifestyle, and internal chemistry. To imagine that one dietary model could nourish every person equally is to ignore the intricate variability of human biology.

For over a century, diet trends have come and gone. From grapefruit diets and meal replacements to high-protein regimens and supplement-heavy plans. Yet despite the explosion of nutritional advice, we are now living in the era of the most widespread obesity in modern history. Something is amiss.

In my own journey through health and performance—especially as I've aged—I've seen how easy it is to disconnect from our internal wisdom. We chase after programs, experts, and formulas, often bypassing the most powerful guide we have: our inner voice. Long-lasting change doesn't come from outsourcing our choices. It begins with tuning in to our own physiology.

Let me pose a question: if five people eat the same meal—the same salad, the same steak, from the same cow—will each person receive the same nutrients in the same proportions?

The answer is no.

What we absorb from our food is shaped by a multitude of factors, broadly divided into two categories: internal and external.

INTERNAL FACTORS: THE MACHINERY OF NUTRIENT ABSORPTION

- Digestion is the mechanical and chemical breakdown of food into smaller components that can be absorbed by the body.
- Assimilation is the process through which the body absorbs nutrients from digested food, enables the construction and repair of cells, ultimately leading to the formation of the body's fluids and tissues.

- Metabolism refers to all chemical reactions in the body that convert food into energy and building blocks for growth, repair, and maintenance.
- Elimination is the removal of indigestible substances and metabolic waste from the body, primarily through feces and urine.

These functions do not operate the same way in every person. Two individuals may consume the same meal and absorb vastly different amounts of fats, proteins, carbohydrates, and micronutrients. We are not machines—our physiological responses are deeply personal and ever-changing.

EXTERNAL FACTORS: THE WEIGHT OF MODERN LIFE

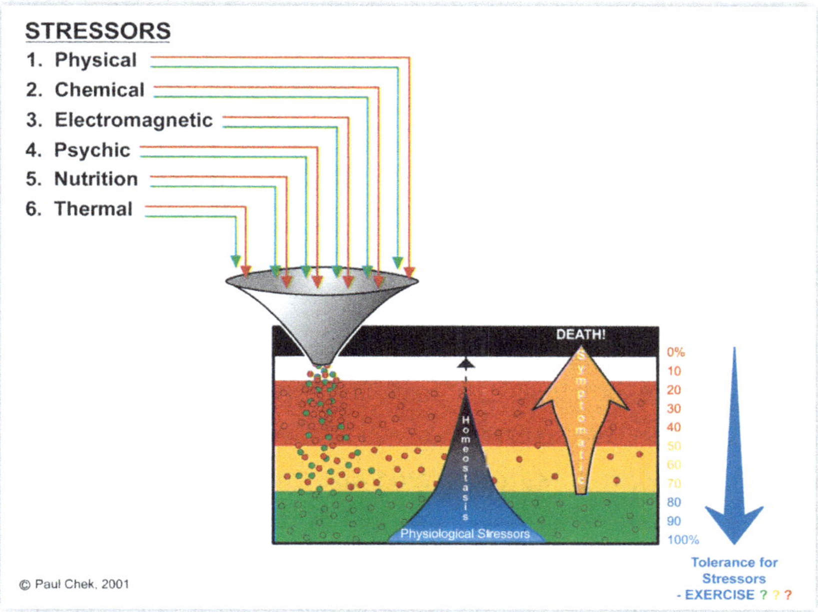

Figure 1: Chek, P. (2004). *How to Eat, Move, and Be Healthy!* CHEK Institute.

External stressors play a critical role in how we digest and utilize food. The model shown in Figure 1 outlines six major stress categories:

1. Physical factors such as exercise, poor posture, or injuries.
2. Chemical factors include environmental chemicals, food additives, and vitamins.
3. Electromagnetic factors primarily originate from natural sunlight, but contemporary stressors include artificial lighting and electronic devices.
4. Psychic stressors include mental and emotional factors.
5. Nutritional stressors result from consuming potentially harmful substances like alcohol, caffeine, and other suboptimal foods.
6. Thermal stressors are of utmost importance. The body's most energy-intensive system, the thermoregulatory system, is perpetually engaged. Conditions like inflammation or hypothyroidism increase its workload.

Certain stressors are essential for maintaining health (indicated by green arrows), while others are detrimental to the body (indicated by red arrows). However, excessive levels of these stressors, such as excessive exercise, can lead to adverse outcomes.

For instance, when negative stressors are low, we stay in the green zone and our response to exercise can be positive. However, when the level of negative stressors increases, we enter the yellow zone and potentially progress to the red zone over time or if the level of stressors becomes excessive. As a result, we become increasingly symptomatic. The more symptomatic we become, our tolerance for exercise and other stress lowers, and consequently the closer we approach death.

Stress is the most common cause of disrupted digestion, elimination, body pain, and mental emotional imbalance in general, and each of us perceive it uniquely. Stress perception is highly individual. Would you and LeBron James feel the same level of stress going into a game 7 championship final?

THE BIOAVAILABILITY PUZZLE

Bioavailability can differ greatly from person to person, even when they eat the same meal. This becomes especially clear when we look at how individual nutrient needs vary so widely. A great book that explores this in depth is *Biochemical Individuality* by Roger Williams.

Someone deficient in magnesium may extract more from food containing it. Another person, already well-nourished, may absorb little. What's nourishing for one may be depleting for another.

BIOAVAILABILITY

The body's ability to absorb and use nutrients.

As a former soldier accustomed to *Meals Ready to Eat (MREs)*, I know firsthand how these industrially-produced rations meet only the bare minimum for survival. For someone raised on nutrient-dense, whole foods, MREs feel like a downgrade. Yet to a person with limited food access, they might represent a nutritional step forward. Context matters.

DIGESTIVE CAPACITY: USE IT OR LOSE IT

Digestion requires effort. The more processed a food is, the less work your body must do to digest it and the weaker your digestive system becomes over time. Consuming soft, pre-digested foods like protein powders or heavily fortified bars can be as compromising as wearing a back brace for too long. Like underused muscles, the gut begins to atrophy.

> **DIGESTION**
>
> The process by which your body breaks down food into smaller pieces and converts it into nutrients. These can then be absorbed and used for growth, repair and energy.

Laxatives tell the same story. Rely on them too often, and the body forgets how to move its bowels naturally. True health demands engagement—not shortcuts.

WHAT IS HOLISM?

Whole foods provide the body with complete systems of nutrition that can bring about harmony in our physiology. In many ways, harmony is another word for health.

Every food carries its own energy. That energy has a "charge" or quality. Traditional philosophies describe this as yin and yang:

- **Yang** energy is outward, active, and consuming. Think of the sun—its nuclear core burns as it sends energy and light in every direction. Yang is associated with activity, expenditure, and often with masculine qualities.

- **Yin** energy is inward, receptive, and conserving. It's connected to rest, repair, the parasympathetic nervous system, and feminine qualities. Yin builds and restores resources.

Too much yang—too much output—leads to depletion. Without yin to restore balance, the body cannot sustain its power. A simple example is water balance: if you sweat but don't drink, you end up depleted and dehydrated. The same principle applies to training, work, or emotional stress—if resources aren't replenished with sound nutrition, performance and vitality decline.

Living foods carry more energetic "charge" than processed foods. Raw foods often hold more life-force than cooked foods. By listening closely to your body, you can sense which foods bring you back into balance.

Food is more than calories—it's information. Just as a stop sign tells us to press the brakes, the body reads food signals and makes changes in energy use, repair, and growth. Healthy cravings are your body's way of asking for specific types of energy and information to restore equilibrium.

Imbalance usually appears in two forms: excesses and deficiencies.

- **Excess** comes from too much of a food, vitamin, or supplement—or from harmful exposures such as additives, preservatives, pesticides, or artificial colorings.
- **Deficiency** arises when the body's needs are not met due to lack of awareness or poor diet choices.

A clear example of excess is the overconsumption of what I call "The Four White Devils":

1. White flour
2. White sugar
3. White processed table salt
4. Pasteurized dairy

These foods contribute to acidity in the body. To buffer excess acidity, the body often pulls calcium from its own reserves. Over time, this can weaken bones and lead to osteoporosis.

A long-term study published in the American Journal of Clinical Nutrition (2006) tracked over 2,500 men and women. It found women who drank three or more cola-based sodas daily had about 4 % lower bone mineral density (BMD) in the hip compared to non-drinkers. It is thought that excess sugar made their blood too acidic. The body, trying to buffer the acid, pulled calcium from the bones.

This is what we mean by a *deficiency disease*—illness created not because food is absent, but because the wrong foods deplete essential nutrients.

Holism reminds us that health is not about isolated nutrients or single solutions. It is about the whole: whole foods, living foods, balance between yin and yang, and awareness of how what we eat informs and energizes the body. When we see food as energy and information, we become more capable of creating lasting harmony within ourselves.

To thrive, we must do more than follow the next diet trend. We must listen deeply. Food is energy, information, and medicine. By tuning in to our inner signals, choosing living foods, and honoring our unique biology, we take the first step toward true wellness.

Let's begin this journey not with rigid rules, but with awareness—and a willingness to see food not as an enemy or savior, but as a partner in our personal evolution.

CHAPTER 2

THE LOST LEGENDS OF FOOD SCIENCE & WHAT THEY TAUGHT US

"Every truth passes through three stages:
First, it is ridiculed. Second, it is violently opposed.
Third, it is accepted as being self-evident."

~ Arthur Schopenhauer

Throughout the late 19th and early 20th centuries, a handful of pioneering physicians and researchers uncovered a truth that modern science continues to confirm: diet is one of the most powerful determinants of human health. They documented how processed, industrial foods fostered disease, while whole, traditional diets sustained life, strength, and longevity. Their findings remain strikingly relevant today, reminding us that the choices we make at the table ripple through our bodies, minds, and even into future generations.

SIR ROBERT MCCARRISON

Sir Robert McCarrison (1878–1960) was a pioneering British physician and nutritionist whose research revealed the profound influence of diet on health and longevity. His work gained urgency during the World Wars, when more than 40% of military recruits were rejected for service due to malnutrition. This posed a national security concern, since young men aged 17 to 25, who should have been in their physical prime, were among the least fit for duty.

In his investigations, McCarrison examined dietary habits across cultures and identified the Hunza people of northern India as among the healthiest and longest-lived. Their diet was simple but nutrient-dense, consisting of unleavened bread made from freshly ground wheat, dairy products such as fresh milk, butter, curds, and buttermilk, along with an abundance of leafy greens, root vegetables like potatoes and carrots, seasonal fruits, and, when available, modest portions of meat.

To test the effects of this diet scientifically, McCarrison conducted a two-year experiment with roughly 1,600 rats—a span comparable to about 55 human years. Remarkably, at the end of the study, none of the rats fed the Hunza diet exhibited disease. Deaths occurred only from natural aging, maternal mortality was absent, and the animals remained vigorous throughout their lives.

He then repeated the experiment with another 1,600 rats, this time replicating the typical English diet of the early 20th century. This diet was dominated by white bread, margarine, tinned meats, boiled vegetables, inexpensive canned goods, jam, tea, sugar, and only small amounts of milk. The contrast was stark. These rats grew poorly, developed illnesses, and displayed disturbed behavior. By the 16th day, stronger rats began attacking and consuming weaker ones, forcing researchers to separate them into individual cages.

The diseased rats mostly suffered from lung, stomach, and intestinal disorders, as well as neurological conditions. Strikingly, the prevalence of these illnesses mirrored the patterns observed among the English population of the time, underscoring McCarrison's conclusion that diet plays a decisive role not only in physical health but also in mental and emotional stability.

In later studies, summarized in his 1936 *Cantor Lectures*, McCarrison further explored the relationship between diet, disease, and behavior by testing a variety of dietary compositions on rats, Rats were fed a basal diet that consisted of 20 parts meat residue, 60 parts purified starch, 8 parts olive oil, 5 parts salt mixture and 7 parts indigestible foodstuffs. The results of that diet can be seen in the Figure 2. In 14 days they lost weight and were paralyzed, with most of them dying of beri-beri in 27-47 days!

These experiments consistently reinforced his central insight: that the quality of food profoundly shapes both the vitality of the body and the balance of the mind.

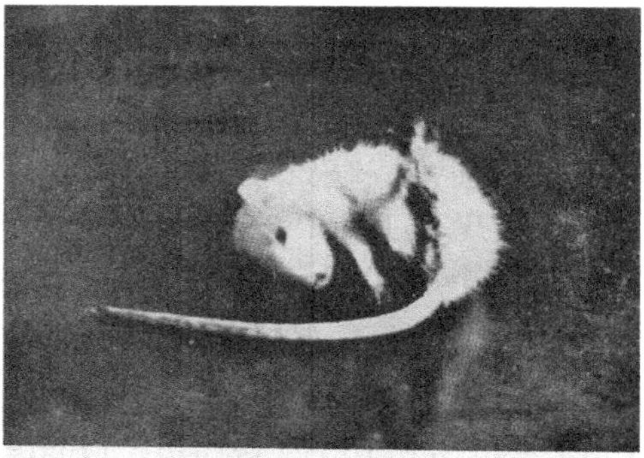

XIV. BASAL DIET RAT
who, though he had all the calories and body-building foods he needed, died from want of vitamins

Figure 2: Picton, L. J. (1956). *Thoughts on Feeding.* Faber and Faber.

DR. JOHN KELLOGG

Dr. John Harvey Kellogg (1852–1943) was an American medical doctor, nutritionist, and inventor. He is best known for his role in creating corn flakes.

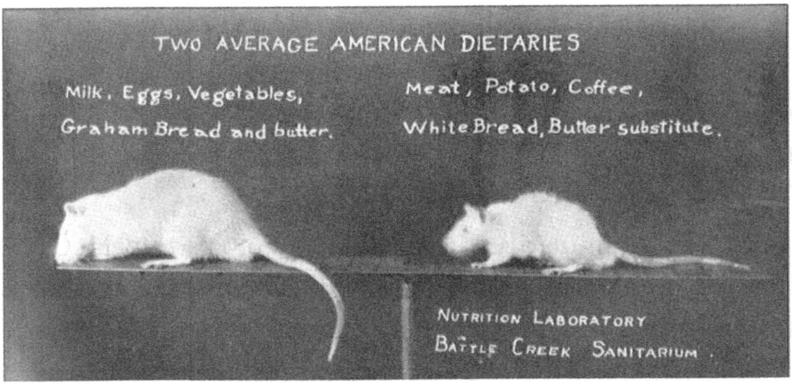

Figure 3: Richardson, I. D. (1932). *Diet and disease*. ME-NA Vita Co.

Kellogg did an experiment where he fed mice two different diets. The mouse on the left was fed milk, eggs, vegetables, Graham (whole wheat) bread, and butter. The mouse on the right, the little scrawny one, got meat, potato (no other vegetables), white bread, butter substitute and coffee.

What surprised me most was discovering that this study, conducted in 1932, used a butter substitute. I had not realized that such a product even existed at that time, and it was only through this research that I learned it had already been invented.

FRANCIS MARION POTTENGER SR., M.D.

Francis Marion Pottenger Sr., M.D. (1869–1960), was an American physician and researcher whose work spanned tuberculosis treatment, the autonomic nervous system, and nutritional science. In 1919, he published *Symptoms of Visceral Disease*, a landmark text that examined how the nervous system influences organ function, with particular emphasis on the adrenal glands. More than a century later, his research remains influential, underscoring its lasting significance.

Between 1932 and 1942, Pottenger conducted one of the most well-known nutritional experiments of the twentieth century. Originally initiated during his studies on adrenal extracts for tuberculosis patients, the project evolved into a decade-long exploration of how diet shapes health across multiple generations of cats. The results were published in his book, *Pottenger's Cats*.

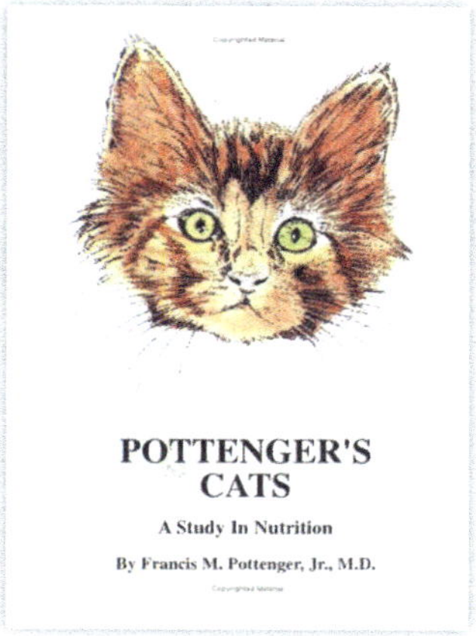

The design was straightforward: one group of cats was fed a natural diet of raw meat, raw milk, and cod liver oil, while another group received cooked meat and pasteurized milk. The outcomes, however, were anything but ordinary.

Cats nourished with raw, unprocessed foods thrived. They developed strong immune systems, healthy bone structures, glossy coats, and displayed normal reproductive patterns and behaviors. In stark contrast, the cats consuming cooked meat and pasteurized milk experienced progressive degeneration. Their health problems included weakened immunity, higher rates of infections and allergies, bone deformities and arthritis, and serious reproductive issues such as miscarriages and infertility. Behavioral disturbances also emerged, with cats becoming either aggressive or lethargic. Alarmingly, reproductive decline was evident within just a few generations: the first generation showed a 25% miscarriage rate, which rose to 70% in the second. By the third generation, the cats were infertile and died prematurely, effectively ending the lineage.

Pottenger's findings drew attention to the role of enzymes in food. Pasteurization, while extending the shelf life of milk by halting enzymatic activity, also eliminated the natural enzymes needed for proper digestion and assimilation. As a result, the body was forced to supply these enzymes itself, leading to gradual depletion. This concern was echoed by biochemist Ehrenfried Pfeiffer in 1957, who observed that by the age of 32 to 35, many individuals were already enzyme-deficient with severely compromised liver function. Pfeiffer argued that this deficiency reflected a dangerous misconception underlying industrialized food production.

Yet, Pottenger also discovered hope. When malnourished cats were returned to a raw food diet, their health began to recover. Although it required several generations to fully restore vitality, the finding suggested that nutritional damage, while profound, could be reversed over time.

The implications of Pottenger's work resonate powerfully today. In an era marked by rising childhood obesity, early-onset cardiovascular disease, and other chronic conditions, his cat studies serve as a cautionary tale. They remind us that the processed food experiment currently unfolding in human populations mirrors the decline once observed in his laboratory animals. Nutrition, Pottenger's research makes clear, is not simply about calories or convenience; it is a generational determinant of health, vitality, and survival.

DR. WESTON A. PRICE

Dr. Weston A. Price (1870–1948) was a Canadian dentist and pioneering researcher whose work reshaped our understanding of holistic health and nutrition. He devoted his career to studying the connection between diet, dental health, and overall well-being, producing some of the most influential research of the early twentieth century.

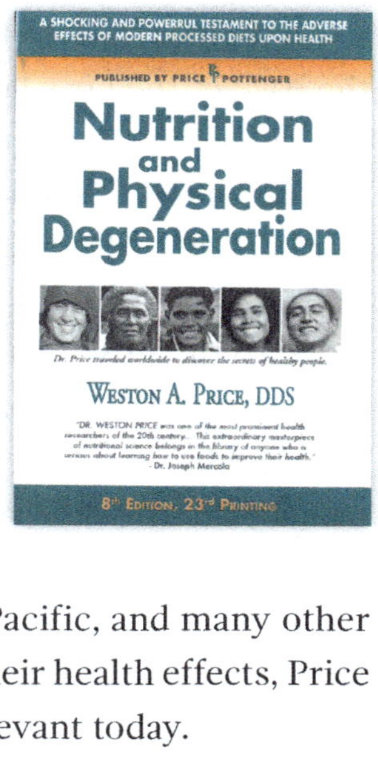

In his seminal book, *Nutrition and Physical Degeneration* (1939), Price documented extensive travels throughout the 1920s and 1930s, during which he studied isolated traditional cultures across the globe. His journeys took him to Switzerland, Scotland, the Arctic, Africa, New Zealand, the South Pacific, and many other regions. By observing indigenous diets and their health effects, Price provided insights that remain profoundly relevant today.

One of his most striking findings was the rapid decline in health when indigenous populations were exposed to "Western" diets dominated by processed foods. Within a single year of dietary change, communities began to experience widespread dental decay, tooth loss, and other signs of degeneration. By contrast, groups that remained unexposed to industrialized foods not only displayed robust health but, in some cases, did not even possess a word for cancer in their languages. For example, Native American tribes in Canada had no historical record of the disease until processed foods were introduced.

Price also studied intergenerational effects. He found that the children of populations exposed to Western foods exhibited profound structural dysfunctions that their genetics could not correct. These changes were most evident in craniofacial development. According to the "rule of thirds," the face should be evenly divided into three equal segments: from the hairline to the eyebrows, the eyebrows to the base of the nose, and the base of the nose to the bottom of the chin. In populations consuming nutrient-deficient diets, this harmony was disrupted. The middle third was often shortened, and the lower third distorted, leading to compromised growth and development.

Price frequently observed that the maxilla (upper jaw) became underdeveloped compared to the mandible (lower jaw). A shortened middle third restricted the airway, impairing breathing and triggering overactivation of the sympathetic nervous system. This, in turn, led to forward head posture and chronic musculoskeletal dysfunction. Such maladaptive growth patterns, Price concluded, occurred when either or both parents were malnourished at the time of conception or during the child's development.

The message of Price's research is clear and timeless: healthy food produces healthy people. His work remains a foundational reference in integrative health, reminding us that nutrition does not merely influence appearance or dental integrity—it determines structural development, resilience against disease, and the vitality of future generations.

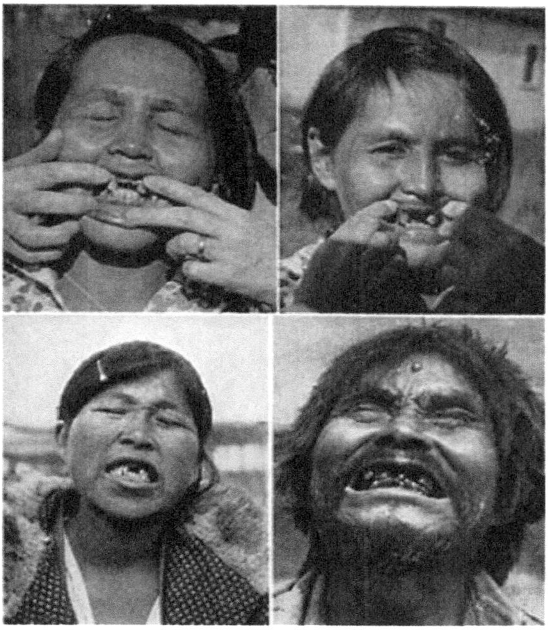

Figure 4: Price, W. A. (2009). *Nutrition and Physical Degeneration: A comparison of primitive and modern diets and their effects* (6th ed.). Price-Pottenger Nutrition Foundation.

WILLIAM L. WOLCOTT

A generation after these pioneering researchers, and building on their body of work, in the late 1970s Bill Wolcott began to develop the concept of Metabolic Typing®. In 1983 he discovered critical new dimensions of the way in which human metabolism is controlled by the oxidative system and the autonomic nervous system. Over the course of the 1980s and 1990s Wolcott made many additional discoveries that continued to transform Metabolic Typing® into a multi-dimensional clinical and academic discipline.

His book, *The Metabolic Typing Diet: Customize Your Diet To: Free Yourself from Food Cravings: Achieve Your Ideal Weight; Enjoy High Energy and Robust Health; Prevent and Reverse Disease*, and his system which creates computer-based, customized "metabolic profiles" for clients and patients, was pivotal in the development of the Primal Pattern® Eating system.

CHAPTER 3

THE PRIMAL PATTERN® DIET

"Food and water should *always* be your first medicine."
~ Hippocrates

Through years of studying the pioneers of nutritional research in the 20th century, such as Sir Robert McCarrison, Dr. John Kellogg, Francis Pottenger, M.D., Weston Price, D.D.S., Royal Lee, D.D.S., Roger Williams, Ph.D and William Wolcott, I discoverd a consistent theme emering. While people can be categorized into different metabolic types, the single most important influence on dietary patterns across human history has been **availability**. In other words, what people eat is largely determined by what their environment provides.

Medical researcher Byron Robinson, M.D., provided a fascinating anatomical perspective on this. He is reported to have performed hundreds of dissections—possibly as many as 650—to determine whether intestinal length varied among individuals from different regions and dietary traditions. His findings were striking. Populations that relied heavily on plant foods, with limited access to animal flesh, often had intestinal tracts nearly twice as long as those who primarily consumed meat. By contrast, groups such as the Inuit, whose diets consist almost entirely of flesh foods, fat, and protein, exhibited notably shorter digestive tracts.

These adaptations reflect the environments in which these populations lived. The Inuit survive in Arctic conditions where 90 percent of the diet must come from animal protein and fat due to the absence of plant foods. Equatorial populations, on the other hand, enjoy year-round access to abundant plant life, supported by warm climates and the absence of freezing winters. Their diets are therefore more plant-based, with animal foods included when available. Over generations, these environments shaped not only dietary patterns but also genetic adaptations, creating a natural alignment between physiology and food sources.

Clinical practice confirms this principle. Many individuals with European ancestry, or those naturally inclined toward protein-rich diets, often struggle when adopting vegetarian or raw food regimens. Their bodies are simply less efficient at extracting nutrients—particularly proteins and other key elements—from high-fiber plant foods. This does not mean vegetarian diets cannot be healthful, but it underscores the reality that such approaches demand thoughtful application and may not suit everyone or every genetic variation.

FINDING YOUR PRIMAL PATTERN® DIET TYPE

To make these distinctions practical, I have simplified dietary tendencies into three primary categories, which I call **Primal Pattern® Diet Types**. These categories reflect both ancestral heritage and genetic design:

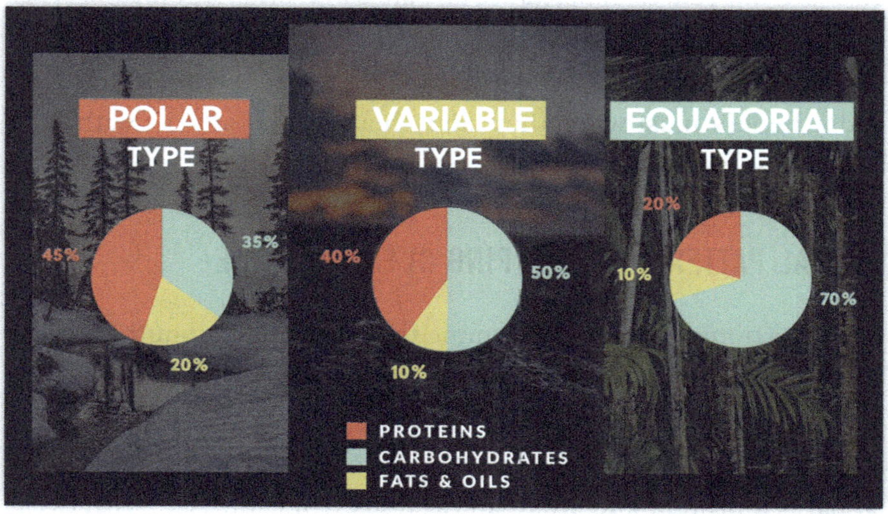

- **Polar Type**—Best suited for those with ancestry in colder climates, Polar Types require higher amounts of fat and protein to thrive. Their physiology favors dense, energy-rich animal foods.
- **Equatorial Type**—Adapted to tropical and subtropical climates, Equatorial Types naturally gravitate toward diets rich in fruits, vegetables, and plant-based staples. Animal foods are included when available but are not the central feature of their nutrition. For example, **Indigenous Australians** living inland in desert environments often relied predominantly on plant foods because of limited access to large game.

- **Variable Type**—Individuals with mixed ancestry fall into this category. They demonstrate greater flexibility and can thrive on diets that include substantial amounts of either plant or animal foods. Their needs often shift more dynamically than those of Polar or Equatorial Types.

In short, our genetic inheritance and ancestral origins guide the types of foods we are best equipped to process. Just as the Inuit cannot sustain themselves on a plant-based diet in the Arctic, individuals today benefit most when they align their eating patterns with their Primal Pattern® Type.

PRIMAL PATTERN® DIET TYPING QUESTIONNAIRE

The questionnaire helps determine the optimal macronutrient ratio (protein to carbohydrate to fat) to fine-tune your body's feedback mechanisms.

What is a protein and what isn't? Foods from sources "with eyes" (cows, sheep, birds, fish) are higher in fats and proteins, which often occur together. Conversely, foods from sources "without eyes" (vegetables, fruits, cereals) are higher in carbohydrates and lower in fats and proteins. However, there are exceptions like nuts, seeds, and avocados, which are high in fat despite lacking eyes.

When answering the questions, circle the answer that best describes your current feelings, not your ideal eating habits! If none of the answers align with your current feelings for a particular question, simply skip it. If you find that answer A suits you some days (like in the morning, but not in the evening), and answer B suits you on other days, you can

MACRONUTRIENTS

These are essential nutrients that the body needs in large quantities to provide energy and support growth and development. They include:

Carbohydrates to provide energy, regulate blood sugar levels, and support gut health.

Proteins to build and repair tissues, support immune function, and regulate hormones.

Fats to store energy, protect organs, and transport vitamins and minerals.

circle both. However, ensure that the answers refer to your feelings on any given day, not over a period of more than 24 hours.

1. I sleep best:
   - **A.** when I eat a snack high in protein and fat 1-2 hours before going to sleep.
   - **B.** when I eat a snack higher in carbohydrates 3-4 hours before going to sleep.

2. I sleep best if:
   - **A.** my dinner is composed of mainly meat with some vegetables or other carbohydrates.
   - **B.** my dinner is composed mainly of vegetables or other carbohydrates and a comparatively small serving of meat.

3. I sleep best and wake up feeling rested:
   A. if I don't eat sweet deserts like cakes, candy, or cookies. If I eat a rich desert that is not overly sweet, such as high-quality full-fat ice cream, I tend to sleep okay.
   B. if I occasionally eat a sweet desert before I go to bed.

4. After vigorous exercise, I feel best when I consume:
   A. foods or drinks with higher protein and/or fat content, such as a high-protein shake.
   B. foods or drinks higher in carbohydrates (sweeter), such as Gatorade.

5. I do best—maintain mental clarity and a sense of well-being for up to 4 hours after a meal—when I eat:
   A. a meat-based meal containing heavier meats such as chicken legs, roast beef, and salmon, with a smaller portion of carbohydrate.
   B. a carbohydrate-based meal containing vegetables, bread or rice and a small portion of a lighter meat such as chicken breast or white fish.

6. If I am tired and consume sugar or sweet foods such as donuts, candy, or sweetened drinks without significant amounts of fat or protein:
   A. I get a rush of energy, but then I am likely to crash and feel sluggish.
   B. I feel better, and my energy levels are restored until my next meal.

7. Which statement best describes your disposition toward food in general:
   A. I love food and live to eat!
   B. I do not fuss over food, and I eat to live.

8. I often:

A. add salt to my foods.

B. find that foods are too salty for my liking.

9. Instinctually, I prefer to eat:

A. dark meat, such as the chicken or turkey legs and thighs over the white breast meat.

B. light meat such as the chicken or turkey breast over the dark leg and thigh meat.

10. Which list of fish most appeals to you?

A. anchovies, caviar, herring, mussels, sardines, abalone, clams, crab, crayfish, lobster, mackerel, octopus, oysters, salmon, scallops, shrimp, snail, squid, tuna (dark meat).

B. white fish, catfish, cod, flounder, haddock, perch, scrod, sole, trout, tuna (white), turbot.

11. When eating dairy products, I feel best after eating:

A. richer, full fat yogurts and cheeses or desserts.

B. lighter, low fat yogurts and cheeses or desserts.

12. Regarding snacking:

A. I tend to do better when I snack between meals or eat more smaller meals throughout the day.

B. I tend to last between meals without snacking.

13. Which describes the way you instinctively prefer to start your day to feel your best and to have the most energy?

A. Eating a large breakfast that includes protein and fat, such as eggs with sausage or bacon.

B. Eating a light breakfast such as cereal, fruit, yogurt, breads and possibly some eggs.

14. Which characteristics best describe you:

A. In general, I digest food well, have an appetite for proteins, feel good when eating fats or fatty foods, am more muscular or inclined to gain muscle or strength easily.

B. I have a lean build, prefer light meats and lower-fat foods, and am more inclined toward endurance athletics.

Total A answers: ______
Total B answers: ______

To score your test, add the questions you circled A and the number you circled B.

- If your number of A answers is three or more than B answers, you are a Polar Type.
- If your number of A and B answers are tied or within two of each other, you are a Variable Type.
- If your number of B answers is three or more than A answers, you are an Equatorial Type.

FREE BONUS 1

Don't forget, you can also complete your questionnaire online and receive coaching tips based on your results! Simply scan the QR code, follow the instructions, and your results will be emailed to you.

SUMMARY ON PRIMAL PATTERN® DIET TYPES

Polar Type

- Polar Types thrive on consuming more protein, so you'll notice that they naturally gravitate towards animal meats, as they feel their bodies are best nourished by them.
- This preference is often inherited from ancestors who lived in the polar regions of the planet. Consider the fact that growing vegetables in the snow is impossible. Therefore, they relied on consuming meat, which provided them with some vegetable matter from the bellies of the animals they consumed.
- The typical ratio of animal to plant consumption is approximately 2 to 1. Consequently, when you examine your plate, you'll observe that it will contain twice as much meat or fish as vegetables.

Equatorial Type

- Equatorial Types typically have ancestors who lived near the Equator. In this region, there was more sunlight, which allowed for the cultivation of a wider variety of vegetables. Consequently, due to the extreme heat, there was a scarcity of animals. While animals were consumed when available, their populations were significantly lower compared to other regions.
- The typical ratio of animal to plant consumption is approximately 1 to 2.

Variable Type

- These are the types that are usually created when nationalities integrate with each other. For instance, perhaps your

grandfather came from Canada, and your grandmother was from South America.
- The typical ratio of animal to plant consumption is approximately 1 to 1. However, it's more dynamic than that.
- Variable Type individuals require specific dietary adjustments as their protein and vegetable needs can fluctuate throughout the day.

Testing provides a starting point but shouldn't be considered a fixed prescription. For example, if you suffer from symptoms such as constipation, bloating, or reduced energy after eating a high-protein meal, it's essential to increase your vegetable intake. As you gain clarity and begin to understand what your body is telling you it needs, you'll realize how to tweak your dietary needs, like consuming one egg instead of two or one chicken breast instead of two. It may not sound like a big deal, but it's important to recognize these subtleties.

Your diet changes are also based on temperature and activity level, especially for females during their menstrual cycle. For instance, when it's hot outside, you may crave raw vegetables with some meat or fish, and consuming too much meat may make you hotter or more lethargic. On the other hand, when it's cold, you may prefer a hearty stew with ample protein. Therefore, it's crucial to pay close attention and monitor both your meals, and your reaction to the food carefully.

Often, when experiencing stress, the stomach constricts, becoming tight and making digestion challenging. Consequently, consuming something like a large portion of chicken for lunch or breakfast can lead to discomfort. It is advisable to approach meal planning on a meal-by-meal basis. Before each meal, assess your actual hunger levels and determine the appropriate portion size. If you stick rigidly to a set meal plan, without monitoring your responses and symptoms, you may find yourself suffering from excessive bloating by dinner time!

At times, it is necessary to acknowledge that certain actions may not align with one's current needs. Recognizing and honoring these needs is a crucial step in the personal development process. Further chapters will provide guidance on developing these essential skills.

CHAPTER 4

FROM SOIL HEALTH TO HUMAN HEALTH: THE ORGANIC LINK

"The real wealth of the Nation lies in the resources of the earth—soil, water, forests, minerals, and wildlife."

~ Rachel Carson

THE ORGANIC CLOSED CYCLE

When we talk about food quality, one essential truth stands above all: **life sustains life.**

Healthy food begins not in the supermarket or even in the farmer's field, but deep in the soil. As shown in Figure 5, the process starts with humus, the dark, nutrient-rich material formed from fallen leaves, animal waste, and plant matter. This humus is far more than "dirt." It

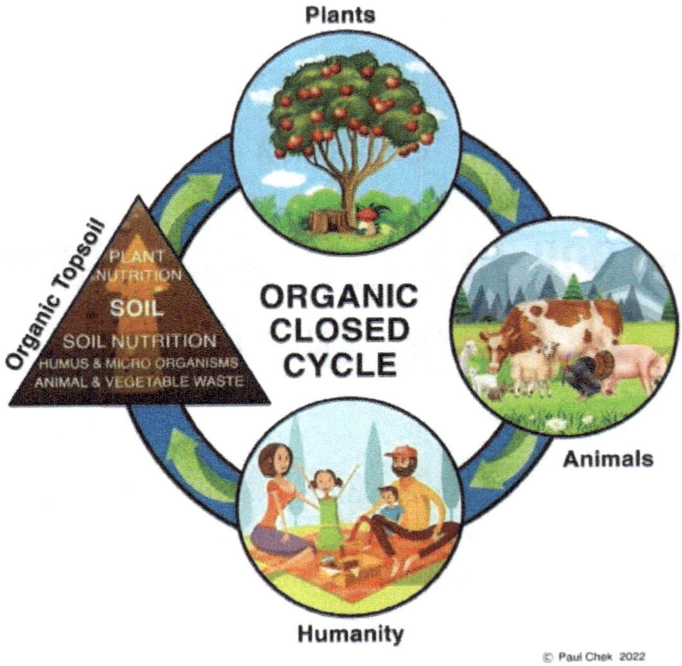

Figure 5: The Organic Closed Cycle, taken from The Master Key online course at myspiritgym.com (Chek, 2024).

is the foundation of a living ecosystem teeming with microorganisms uniquely adapted to their soil environment.

These microbes transform raw organic material into a vibrant, crumb-like soil structure. In doing so, they capture sunlight, earth energy, and the subtle forces of nature, turning soil into a living, breathing system. Plants and animals contribute waste back into this cycle, which in turn nourishes the microorganisms, completing an endless loop of renewal.

True fertilization, then, is not about dumping chemicals into the ground. It is about **feeding the soil community.** When the microbial world thrives, soil maintains its temperature, supports healthy plant growth, and generates the complex nutrients necessary for life itself.

Unfortunately, industrial agriculture has disrupted this natural balance. Chemical fertilizers and pesticides may force crops to grow, but they do so by weakening or destroying the very microorganisms that make soil fertile. Without them, soil becomes depleted, plants lose vitality, animals grow sick, and humans who depend on them inevitably feel the consequences. Taking synthetic vitamins to make up for these losses is like taking aspirin for a persistent headache; it masks the problem without addressing the root cause.

The real solution is simple, yet profound: **care for the source.** By supporting local organic farmers and growers who enrich the soil instead of stripping it, we restore the foundation of health for plants, animals, and people. When we align with nature's wisdom, rather than fight against it, we safeguard not only the vitality of our food but also the health and sustainability of generations to come.

In contrast to the Organic Closed Cycle, Figure 6 reminds us of a sobering truth: modern farming has created a food system that often works against health rather than for it. Industrial agriculture has degraded the soil, contaminated plants, poisoned animals, and introduced heavy drug use into livestock production. These disruptions ripple through the food chain. Humans eat the plants and animals raised in these conditions, and in doing so, ingest residues of toxins, weakened nutrients, and metabolic distortions. The result is reflected in today's skyrocketing rates of chronic disease, obesity, anxiety, depression, and even suicide—the highest in recorded medical history.

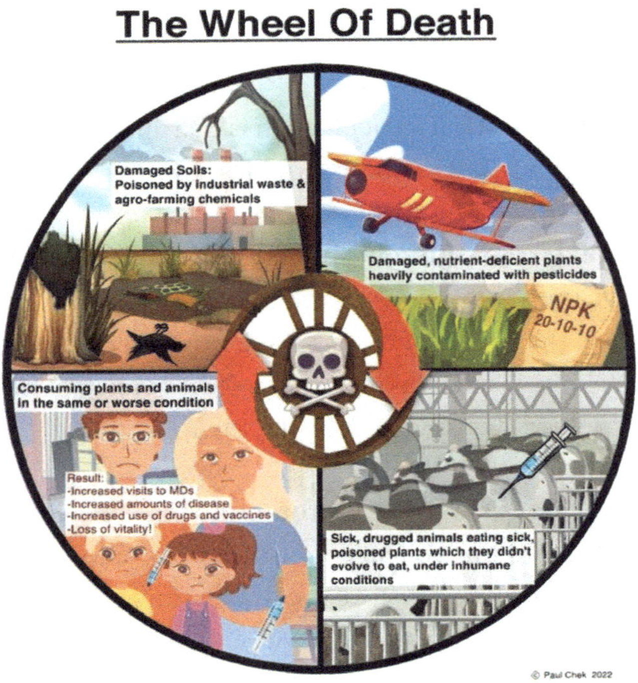
The Wheel Of Death
Damaged Soils:
Poisoned by industrial waste &
agro-farming chemicals
Damaged, nutrient-deficient plants
heavily contaminated with pesticides
NPK
20-10-10
Consuming plants and animals
in the same or worse condition
Result:
-Increased visits to MDs
-Increased amounts of disease
-Increased use of drugs and vaccines
-Loss of vitality!
Sick, drugged animals eating sick,
poisoned plants which they didn't
evolve to eat, under inhumane
conditions
© Paul Chek 2022

Figure 6: The Wheel of Death, taken from The Master Key online course at myspiritgym.com (Chek, 2024).

WHAT THE SCIENCE SHOWS

In *Nutrition and Biodynamics: Evidence for the Nutritional Superiority of Organic Crops* (Biodynamics, Issue 224), Virginia Worthington, M.S., Sc.D., C.N.S., reviewed 1,230 published studies comparing organic and conventional foods. She found that:

- **56%** of studies favored organic crops.
- **37%** favored conventional crops.
- **7%** found no difference.

At first glance, the 37% figure may seem surprising. How could conventional farming produce "better" results? The answer lies in the influence of large corporations—companies like PepsiCo Inc, Kraft Heinz, and Mars Inc—who have invested heavily in industrial-scale "organic" farming. By shaping certification standards and sponsoring research at agricultural universities, these companies create comparisons that dilute the true advantages of authentic organic food.

Independent reviews tell a clearer story. The British Soil Association analyzed over 400 studies in 2001 (updated in 2007) and found organic foods consistently higher in vitamin C, iron, magnesium, antioxidants, and lower in pesticide residues. Organic meat and dairy contained higher levels of beneficial fatty acids like omega-3s. A 2014 study from Newcastle University showed organic crops had up to **60% more antioxidants** and significantly lower levels of heavy metals such as cadmium and a 2024 study by Rahman et al found that organic food contained higher levels of iron, magnesium and vitamin C.

BEYOND VITAMINS: PHYTONUTRIENTS

Food is more than vitamins and minerals. Plants produce between **5,000-10,000 phytonutrients**—including phenolics, terpenes, alkaloids, and sulfur compounds—that support enzyme activity and human metabolism. Processing destroys many of these delicate compounds, leaving food empty of critical resources. This loss contributes to obesity, metabolic dysfunction, and today's chronic health crises.

Soils rich in microbial life, like those on organic and biodynamic farms, help plants build more complete proteins and higher-quality nutrition. Conventionally-grown plants often fall short.

GRAINS AND THEIR LIMITS

Grains make up nearly half of the average diet, yet modern grains are often nutritionally weak. They lack essential amino acids like lysine, taurine, tryptophan, and arginine—nutrients essential for growth, immunity, metabolism, and mental clarity.

Ehrenfried Pfeiffer, a pioneer of biodynamic agriculture, showed in the 1950s that American grains had lost nutritional density. Conventional grains averaged 12% protein, while biodynamic grains yielded closer to 18%. Ancestral grains were even richer, fueling resilience and growth in ways today's refined flours cannot.

Worse, modern processing introduces anti-nutrients such as phytic acid and increases sugar spikes. Finely milled flour exposes 10,000 times more surface area, causing rapid insulin surges linked to obesity and type 2 diabetes. Whole grains like steel-cut oats digest more slowly, training the digestive system and stabilizing metabolism. Just as muscles weaken without exercise, digestion weakens without robust, whole foods.

THE ANIMAL FACTOR

The same holds true for livestock. Commercial animals are often fed disturbing diets including rendered proteins, bakery waste, industrial oils, and even crops fertilized with sewage sludge. Growth hormones and chemical additives distort protein metabolism, producing nutritionally compromised meat.

Experiments confirm this link between soil, plants, and animals. In *Thoughts on Feeding*, physician Lionel Picton described studies showing that wheat fertilized naturally (with cattle manure) produced healthier animals than wheat grown with chemical fertilizers. Bigger does not mean better; chemically boosted crops and animals may grow larger but often at the cost of vitality and nutritional integrity.

SOIL, FOOD, AND TRUE HEALTH

At the heart of the issue is the soil. When pesticides and chemicals disrupt microbial life, the entire chain of fertility collapses. Worms, microbes, and fungi are not agricultural "extras"; they are the very engines of health. Without them, soil, plants, animals, and people all decline.

Not all "organic" labels are equal. Biodynamic, regenerative farming remains the gold standard, followed by rigorous organic practices. Corporate-controlled certification systems often do little more than market industrial products as "organic." The surest way to secure real food quality is to know your farmer, understand their practices, and support those who work in harmony with natural cycles.

Choosing true organic and biodynamic food is more than a personal health choice. It is a commitment to support the planet, the soil, and the future of humanity.

CHAPTER 5

BEYOND VITAMINS AND CALORIES

"Rowing harder doesn't help if
the boat is headed in the wrong direction."
~ **Kenichi Ohmae**

THE VITAMIN MENTALITY

For more than a hundred years, nutrition in Western culture has been shaped by a medical mindset that prioritizes isolated fixes over whole nourishment. Instead of focusing on food as nature provides it, nutrition was reframed through a reductionist lens—chemicals, compounds, and quick solutions. Few people realize that the first formal nutrition programs in universities were initiated by General Mills. Their goal was not simply scientific discovery, but the promotion of processed food products under the banner of "nutrition science."

From this beginning, the field became deeply intertwined with industry. Even the very concept of "vitamins" was redefined—not as essential parts of whole foods, but as isolated substances that could be extracted, synthesized, and sold either as pills or as fortifications in processed foods.

One of the strongest critics of this approach was Dr. Royal Lee (1895–1967), a dentist, inventor, and nutrition pioneer. Lee insisted that health depended on whole, unprocessed foods. In 1929, he founded *Standard Process*, a company dedicated to producing supplements made from real food concentrates rather than synthetic isolates. His core message was simple but profound: **a vitamin's effectiveness depends on the food matrix it comes with.** Stripped from that natural context, vitamins often do little more than help the body process poor-quality food.

True nutrition, Lee argued, is not about adding pills to a weak diet. It's about eating balanced, nutrient-rich foods that provide the body with the full spectrum of compounds needed for digestion, metabolism, and healing. While supplementation has its place in treating certain deficiencies or toxicities, the deeper problem is that modern farming and processing leave us with food that is calorie-dense but nutrient-poor.

THE IMPORTANCE OF VARIETY AND SEASONALITY

Even those who seek out quality foods can run into problems if their diets are too limited. Variety matters. Nature designed seasonal foods to meet seasonal needs—cooling fruits in summer, grounding roots in winter. Eating seasonally and diversely strengthens resilience, widens nutrient intake, and aligns the body with natural rhythms. Supplements can never fully replace this living, adaptive nourishment.

The lesson is clear: true vitality does not come from bottles of isolated compounds or from processed foods with "added vitamins." It comes from a living relationship with soil, plants, animals, and the cycles of the seasons.

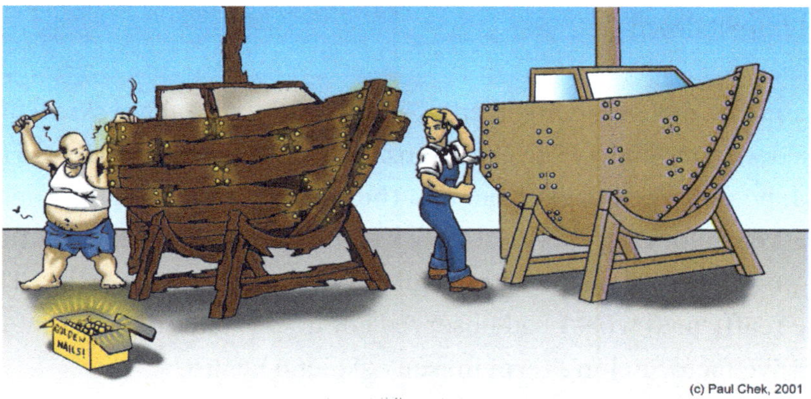

Figure 7: Chek, P. (2004). *How to Eat, Move, and Be Healthy!* CHEK Institute.

To illustrate this, imagine two builders constructing a boat (see Figure 7). One uses poor-quality wood but fastens it with golden nails. The other uses strong, healthy wood with ordinary nails. Which boat would you trust to cross the water? The wood represents food—the foundation. The nails represent vitamins. Without solid material to begin with, no amount of "golden nails" can make a boat seaworthy. Likewise, no supplement can make up for an inferior diet.

As a rehabilitation specialist working with spinal injuries and chronic conditions, I've seen this truth play out thousands of times. Almost all my patients lived on the standard American diet (SAD), a menu of refined and processed foods—what I call SAD *CRAP* (Carbohydrates Refined and Processed).

My father summed it up bluntly: "*You can't make chicken salad out of chicken shit.*" When the body is fed poor materials, it has no choice but to build tissues—bones, cartilage, muscles, nerves—out of those same poor materials. The result is degeneration, dysfunction, and early breakdown.

One memorable case involved a 35-year-old world-class skier diagnosed with multiple disc herniations. When the surgeon reviewed the MRI, he remarked in disbelief that the spine looked more like that of a 75-year-old. Despite the athlete's exceptional physical condition, his poor diet had silently undermined his structural integrity. This case reaffirmed what I had observed countless times before: diet is a decisive factor in long-term musculoskeletal health.

THE CALORIE-COUNTING MENTALITY

Modern culture has layered another problem on top of poor nutrition: an obsession with calories and technology. Fitness trackers, smartwatches, and calorie-counting apps can provide useful feedback on activity and heart rate, but they also come with hidden costs. Overreliance on gadgets dulls self-awareness. Many people forget they can feel their own pulse, sense their breathing, or gauge exertion intuitively—skills that humans developed long before technology.

There is also the issue of constant exposure to Bluetooth and electromagnetic fields. Though rarely discussed, these signals may interfere with subtle biological systems, including cellular communication, the body's energy meridians, and even the energetic flow described in traditions as chakras.

Perhaps the greatest danger of these devices is the illusion of control they create. A person may see that they "burned" 378 calories in a workout, then restrict their next meal to that number. In practice, I have seen these same individuals present with fatigue, poor recovery, and chronic health issues. This is because **food is not just calories, it is *information*.** Restricting intake to match a device readout ignores the body's deeper needs for repair, digestion, hormonal balance, and resilience.

The lesson is clear: health is not a numbers game. It is built on nutrient-dense food, mindful awareness, and respect for the body's complexity.

UNDERSTANDING ENERGY USE

Figure 8 offers a simple way to visualize how the body spends energy:

- The top bowl: Resting Metabolic Rate (RMR). This accounts for 50–70% of daily energy use, covering essentials like breathing, circulation, and heart function.
- The second bowl: Digestion and Elimination. Breaking down food, absorbing nutrients, and processing waste consumes another 5–15% of daily energy.
- The third bowl: Physical Activity. This includes everything from walking to exercise, ranging anywhere from 100 to 1,000 calories or more. This is the only category fitness devices try to measure.

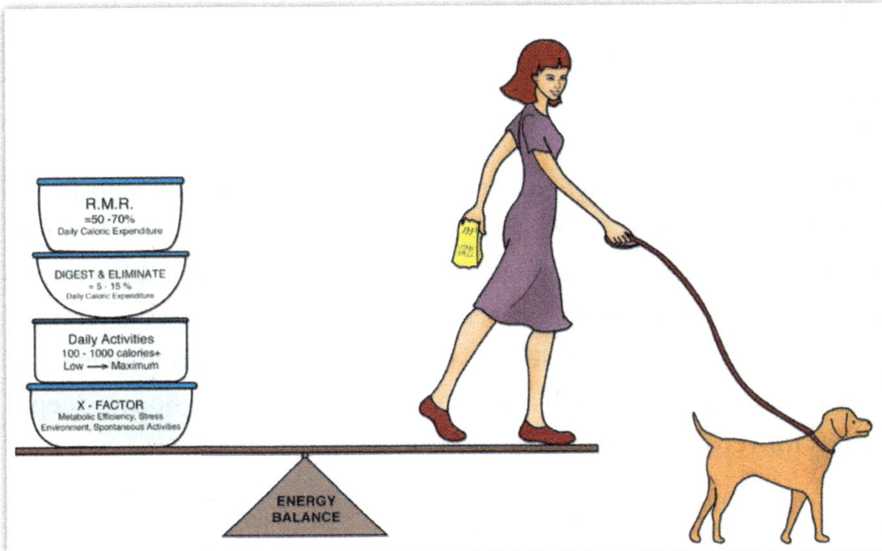
R.M.R.
≈50 -70%
Daily Caloric Expenditure
DIGEST & ELIMINATE
≈ 5 - 15 %
Daily Caloric Expenditure
Daily Activities
100 - 1000 calories+
Low → Maximum
X - FACTOR
Metabolic Efficiency, Stress
Environment, Spontaneous Activities
ENERGY
BALANCE

Figure 8: Chek, P. (2004). *How to Eat, Move, and Be Healthy!* CHEK Institute.

The problem is that when people focus only on "activity calories," they miss the bigger picture. Resting metabolism and digestion are the true energy heavyweights, but they remain invisible to gadgets. This narrow focus reduces human metabolism to a single number—a flawed approach that mirrors the same reductionist thinking behind fad diets and "magic bullet" health products.

DYNAMIC BALANCE, NOT STATIC RULES

Figure 9 illustrates how food is transformed into energy through metabolic pathways, each influencing the hormonal system. The key lesson is this: no principle stands alone. Needs shift constantly depending on environment, stress, and life stage. Health is not a static formula but a living balance, requiring awareness and adaptability.

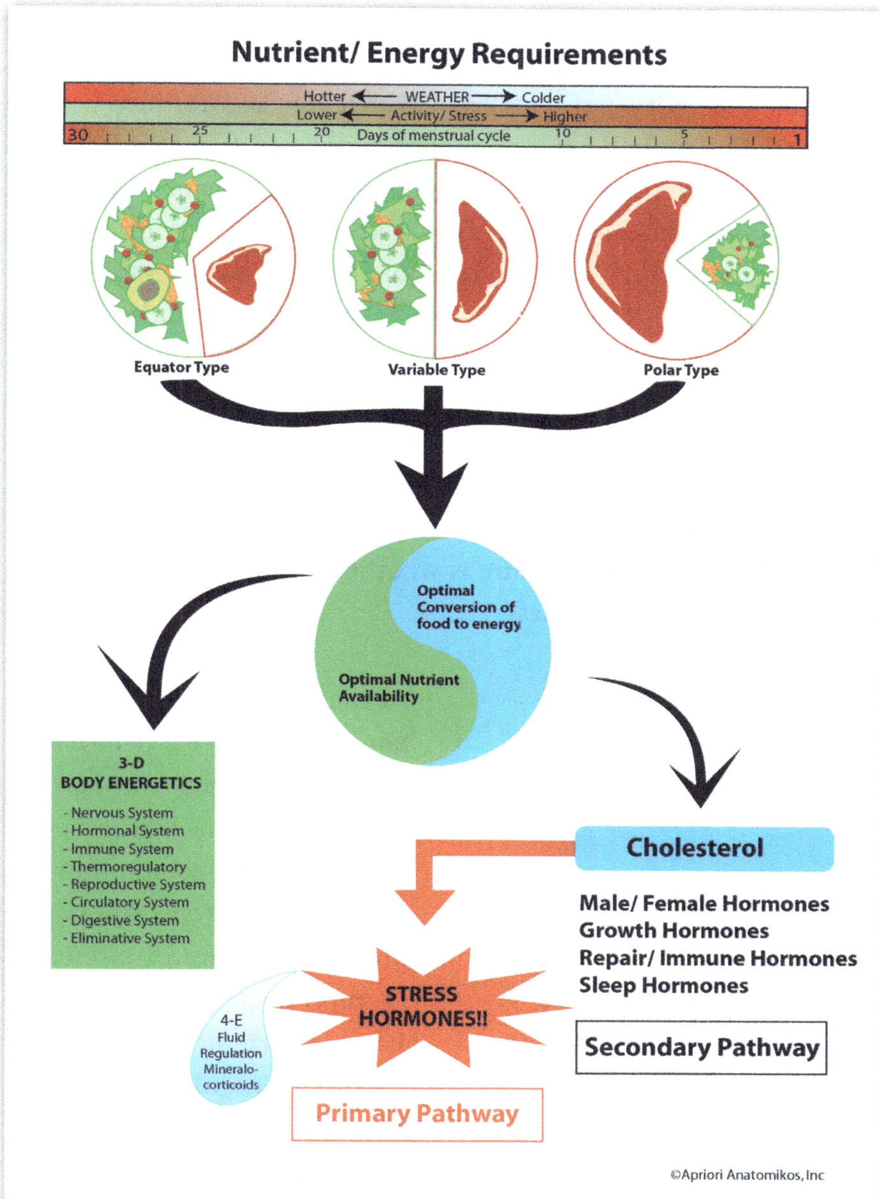

Figure 9: Chek, P. (2004). *How to Eat, Move, and Be Healthy!* CHEK Institute.

For example, weather alters cravings; cold days often drive us toward denser, fattier foods, while hot days call for water-rich fruits and vegetables. Activity and stress also change needs: after heavy resistance training, the body may crave more animal protein, whereas after meditation or light aerobic work, plant-based foods may feel most appropriate. Women often experience stronger cravings for red meat during menstruation, as the body requires nutrients to rebuild blood and uterine tissue. These patterns show that nutrition must respond to the body's signals, not rigid ideology.

One of the greatest mistakes in nutrition is clinging to ideology. Whether it is veganism, vegetarianism, or a carnivore approach, any philosophy can serve for a time, but no single diet suits everyone forever. The only true measure is whether a way of eating supports health, energy, and vitality.

THE KREBS CYCLE (OR CITRIC ACID CYCLE)

This is a series of chemical reactions that are a fundamental part of how cells generate energy from food molecules like glucose. Occurring in the mitochondria of a cell, acetyl-CoA is broken down to release stored energy, producing ATP, NADH, FADH2, and CO2 in the process.

At the deepest level, life is sustained by our ability to turn food into usable energy through the Krebs cycle. This process powers not just movement but the autonomic systems—nervous, hormonal, immune, circulatory, reproductive, and digestive. When nutrient supply falters, these self-regulating systems weaken. Elevated stress in the autonomic nervous system is often the earliest signal of imbalance. Tools such as health appraisal questionnaires, functional medicine assessments, and simple self-awareness can reveal when the body is exceeding its capacity to sustain itself.

Cholesterol, found in flesh foods, butter, and saturated fats, is a precursor to most anabolic hormones, including testosterone and DHEA. These hormones are essential for growth, repair, and resilience. When diets lack sufficient cholesterol, anabolic systems falter. This is particularly common in restrictive plant-based diets.

Genetic differences also matter. As mentioned previously, Byron Robinson, M.D., showed that populations who were historically dependent on plants often evolved longer intestinal tracts to extract more protein from fiber. Populations without these adaptations may struggle to thrive on vegan or vegetarian diets. Comparisons to cows, often cited by plant-based advocates, miss the point—cows have multi-chambered stomachs designed for fiber fermentation. Humans do not.

THE HIDDEN "X FACTOR"

Beneath these measurable layers lies what I call the **X factor**—an element no device can capture. It includes:

- Metabolic efficiency (how well your body uses fuel)
- Environmental stressors (pollution, toxins, EMFs)
- Spontaneous movement (fidgeting, tapping your foot, shifting posture)
- Emotional and mental stress

These factors can shift calorie expenditure dramatically—sometimes from one hour to the next. This is why no calorie-counting device can ever provide a complete picture of metabolism. Human energy balance is dynamic, influenced by body, mind, and environment in ways too complex for a screen to summarize.

For those seeking a deeper dive into this subject, I discuss the intricacies of metabolism in my book *How to Eat, Move, and Be Healthy!* Nutritionist John Berardi has also provided practical insights that contrast with the overly academic theories often taught in universities. His work, like clinical observation, reinforces this truth:

Health cannot be reduced to formulas, numbers, or gadgets. True vitality requires whole food, self-awareness, and a holistic understanding of how the body works.

CHAPTER 6

THE 4 DOCTORS AND THE 6 FOUNDATIONAL PRINCIPLES

"You must begin to think of yourself as becoming the person you want to be."

~ David Viscott

THE LAST 4 DOCTORS YOU'LL EVER NEED

Hippocrates, often honored as the father of medicine, taught that most illnesses could be addressed through three essential physicians: Dr. Diet, the restorer through food and nourishment; Dr. Happiness, the restorer of mind and spirit; and Dr. Quiet, the restorer of rest and recovery. Though he left few details beyond these principles, their simplicity carries timeless wisdom.

Reflecting on this framework in today's world, however, I noticed a gap. Thousands of years ago, people lived physically demanding lives.

Hunting, farming, and daily labor ensured that movement was woven into survival itself. Modern life is different. Inactivity has become one of the greatest threats to health. To adapt Hippocrates' model to contemporary needs, I added a fourth physician: **Dr. Movement**. Together, these four doctors form a complete and functional system for cultivating health and well-being.

Each of the four doctors plays a vital role, though the balance shifts depending on one's circumstances.

- **Dr. Quiet** and **Dr. Diet** are yin in nature. They restore, nourish, and build resilience, which is especially important during times of stress or heavy demand.
- **Dr. Happiness** and **Dr. Movement** bring yang qualities; stimulation, creativity, expression, and engagement with life.

For someone depleted or "too yin"—fatigued, withdrawn, or unmotivated—Dr. Happiness is often the first prescription. Reconnecting with joy, meaning, and purpose can spark recovery. Dr. Movement may also be called, though not through punishing exercise. Instead, gentle practices such as walking, breathwork, tai chi, or yoga can rekindle energy without overwhelming the body. I call this type of exercise *Working-In*, in contrast to the vigors of working-out in a gym, running or riding a bike etc.

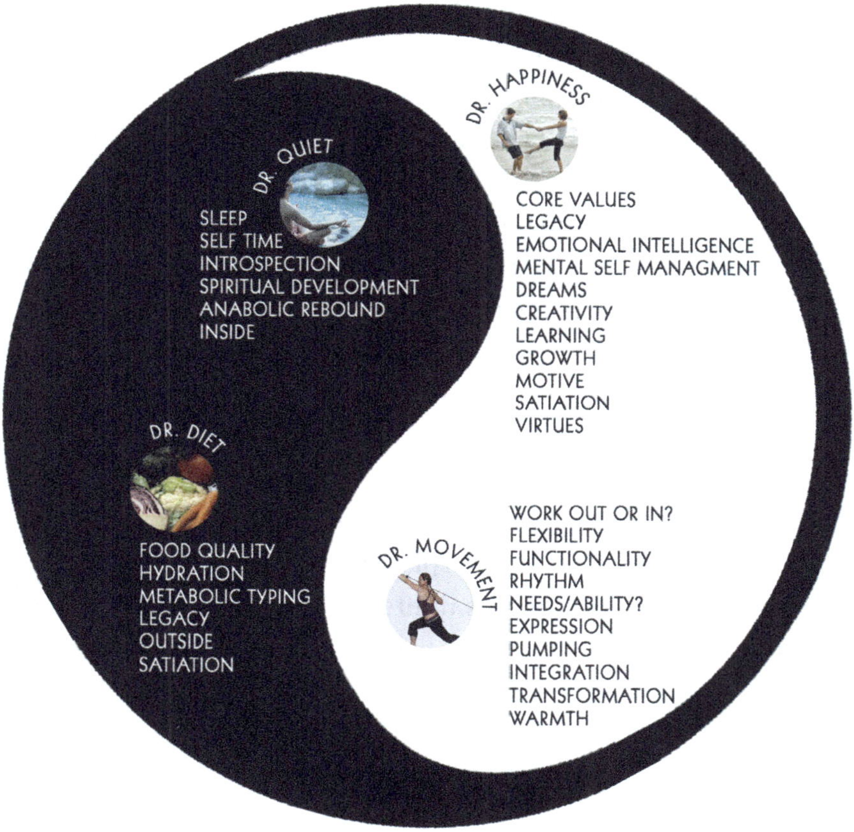
DR. QUIET
SLEEP
SELF TIME
INTROSPECTION
SPIRITUAL DEVELOPMENT
ANABOLIC REBOUND
INSIDE
DR. HAPPINESS
CORE VALUES
LEGACY
EMOTIONAL INTELLIGENCE
MENTAL SELF MANAGMENT
DREAMS
CREATIVITY
LEARNING
GROWTH
MOTIVE
SATIATION
VIRTUES
DR. DIET
FOOD QUALITY
HYDRATION
METABOLIC TYPING
LEGACY
OUTSIDE
SATIATION
DR. MOVEMENT
WORK OUT OR IN?
FLEXIBILITY
FUNCTIONALITY
RHYTHM
NEEDS/ABILITY?
EXPRESSION
PUMPING
INTEGRATION
TRANSFORMATION
WARMTH

Figure 10: Chek, P. (2004). *How to Eat, Move, and Be Healthy!* CHEK Institute.

As illustrated in *Figure 10,* each doctor holds many dimensions.

- **Dr. Quiet** is not merely "taking time out." It includes self-reflection, personal stillness, spiritual practice, and deep recovery from physical training. Quality sleep, for example, is often the result of a day lived with healthy activity. Conversely, insomnia is rarely about an inability to rest; it is often the product of insufficient movement.

Hours spent at a desk leave the body underworked and the mind overstimulated. A simple change, such as rising earlier for a morning walk, moving before meals, or scheduling exercise, allows Dr. Movement to support Dr. Quiet, creating a natural rhythm of rest and renewal.

- **Dr. Diet** nourishes the body's tissues with whole, living foods.
- **Dr. Happiness** keeps the emotional heart engaged. Joy and meaning reduce stress, elevate energy, and reinforce healthy choices.
- **Dr. Movement** expresses life through the body, while also sharpening mental clarity. Movement, in turn, deepens the rest that Dr. Quiet provides.

The 4 Doctors remind us that health does not come from isolated fixes but from the dynamic interplay of nourishment, rest, joy, and movement. At different points in life, we may require more of one and less of another. But to live in balance, all four must be present.

This framework is not about perfection—it's about listening to the body's needs and calling on the right doctor at the right time. Together, they form the most reliable medical team we will ever know.

THE SIX FOUNDATIONAL PRINCIPLES

Building on the wisdom of the 4 Doctors, the CHEK System identifies **six foundational principles** that form the bedrock of health and are the cornerstones of human health and vitality. Three are yin, or restorative in nature: **nutrition, hydration, and sleep.** The other three are yang, or expressive: **breathing, thinking, and movement.** The yin principles provide the raw materials and recovery processes necessary to build and restore the body, while the yang principles express, utilize, and expend that energy in the external world. Together, they create the dynamic balance—homeostasis—that allows life to flourish.

HOMEOSTASIS

The ability of a living organism to maintain a stable internal environment, such as body temperature, blood sugar, and water balance, despite changes in the external environment. It is a self-regulating process that keeps physiological conditions within a narrow range for survival and optimal functioning.

The yin principles remind us that life is fundamentally anabolic: our bodies are constantly rebuilding, repairing, and regenerating. Every year, we replace nearly all of our hundred trillion cells, which means that the quality of our nutrition directly determines the quality of our new tissues. Whole, organic, unprocessed foods provide the building blocks for strong bodies and stable minds. Hydration is equally crucial; nearly every biochemical reaction in the body depends on water, and even slight dehydration can impair mood, cognition, and cellular function. Sleep, often overlooked, is one of the most powerful medicines available, enabling the body to repair itself, regulate hormones, and restore mental clarity. Without adequate nutrition, hydration, and sleep, the body cannot sustain health for long.

The yang principles, by contrast, are the outward expressions of energy and life. Breathing is our most immediate need—without oxygen, life ceases in minutes. It fuels every cell and, when done poorly, can create tension, fatigue, or anxiety. Thinking is another powerful force. Our thoughts shape our emotions, posture, and even physiology, as the body mirrors the state of the mind. With tens of thousands of thoughts generated each day—many of them negative—mental hygiene becomes as important as physical hygiene. Movement is the third yang principle, the visible manifestation of life. From walking and playing to lifting and training, movement transforms the resources of food, water, breath, and rest into external action.

Each principle has both a yin and a yang aspect. For instance, nutrition can be life-giving when balanced, but too much food or the wrong kind creates stress on the body. Hydration sustains life, but over- or under-hydration can become harmful. Sleep restores and rebuilds, but too little or too much can lead to dysfunction. Even breathing, thinking, and moving can become destructive when excessive, shallow, negative, or unbalanced. This is why awareness of both the yin and yang qualities within each principle is so important for creating harmony.

Modern research confirms that 90 to 95 percent of disease does not arise from faulty genetics but from poor application of these very principles. When diet, sleep, water, breath, thought, and movement are compromised, the body's natural balance breaks down and symptoms appear. Conversely, when we align ourselves with these foundations, we create the conditions for energy, vitality, and long-term well-being. They are not quick fixes or isolated hacks, but timeless laws of life that apply to every human being.

Ultimately, the Six Foundational Principles are simple, yet profoundly powerful. They remind us that health is not complicated it is about returning to balance in the most basic human needs. To the degree that we honor these principles and integrate them into daily life, we not only prevent disease but also cultivate strength, clarity, and resilience in body, mind, and spirit. They are the roots from which all other aspects of health and performance grow.

LISTENING TO THE BODY

The body itself is the most reliable research lab. Scientific consensus shifts, but your own physiology offers real-time feedback. Fatigue, cravings, pain, and emotional state all provide clues.

Disease rarely appears overnight. Obesity, cancer, and chronic conditions often build silently over years. The question is whether we pay attention to the signs. Every system—organs, muscles, hormones, digestion, immunity—communicates when out of balance. Suppressing symptoms with drugs or chasing quick fixes ignores the body's wisdom.

Pioneers from Eugen Sandow to Andrew Taylor Still and B.J. Palmer all emphasized the same truth: health is holistic. Muscles, organs, glands, and the nervous system are inseparably linked. Strength and vitality can only be achieved when all systems are in harmony.

THE SPINE-ORGAN CONNECTION

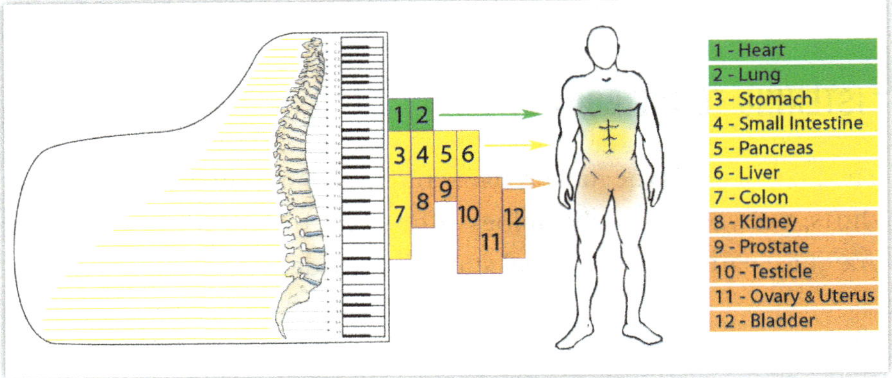

Figure 11: Chek, P. (2004). *How to Eat, Move, and Be Healthy!* CHEK Institute.

The "piano-spine" diagram (*Figure 11*) illustrates how closely the spine and organs are connected. Each organ communicates through the sympathetic nervous system, often expressing dysfunction as musculoskeletal pain. For example, the heart has no sensory neurons of its own—it "borrows" neurons from the left chest, shoulder, and arm. This is why heart trouble often radiates pain into those areas. Many so-called musculoskeletal problems are rooted in gland or organ dysfunction, often tied back to poor diet and lifestyle.

LEARNING TO FEEL TRUE NEEDS

The ultimate lesson of the Six Foundation Principles is that eating—and all health practices—are spiritual acts. True nourishment addresses not just the physical body, but also the emotional and mental bodies. Food cannot fill an empty heart or restless mind.

Emotional starvation often masquerades as hunger, leading to overeating and imbalance.

- The **physical body** thrives on real food and hydration.
- The **emotional body** thrives on love, connection, and healthy expression.
- The **mental body** thrives on awareness, learning, and stimulation.

When one of these is neglected, dysfunction arises. Eating without awareness may temporarily soothe, but it cannot heal deeper needs. Aligning diet and lifestyle with genuine body-mind-spirit requirements transforms eating from a habit into a practice of wholeness.

The Six Foundational Principles remind us: true health is not found in dogma or devices, but in listening to the body, respecting balance, and nourishing all aspects of being.

FREE BONUS 2

Don't settle for gimmicks or quick fixes—claim your FREE ***Flatten Your Abs Forever*** bundle today and get the same proven tools we've used for over 25 years to transform bodies from the inside out. You'll receive two complete video programs—*Flatten Your Abs Forever* and *Gut Health Reset*—revealing how to build a strong, functional core and restore digestive balance for lasting results. Plus, you'll get two powerful e-books: *The Last 4 Doctors You'll Ever Need*, Paul Chek's timeless foundation for health and vitality, and *BIG Bang Workouts*, a high-impact training guide for maximum results in minimal time. All four resources are yours free.

CHAPTER 7

FINE-TUNING: ENERGY & SATIETY IN PRACTICE

"The body is an electrical system, not just a chemical one.
Every healing process begins with a change
in the body's electrical charge."

~ Dr. Robert O. Becker

Refining your diet and lifestyle requires much more than counting calories or balancing macronutrients. **True health depends on a wide spectrum of interrelated factors:** food quality, satiety, energy flow, body temperature, pH balance, mental clarity, emotional stability, motivation, and hydration. Addressing one in isolation provides only partial relief. Thriving requires us to look deeper—to uncover and correct the root causes of imbalance.

To make this clear, I organize these factors into two broad categories: **energy** and **satiety.**

- **Energy** includes flow, temperature, integration, coordination, mental and emotional balance, vision, and motivation.
- **Satiety** includes food quality, the ability to remain full, hydration, and pH balance.

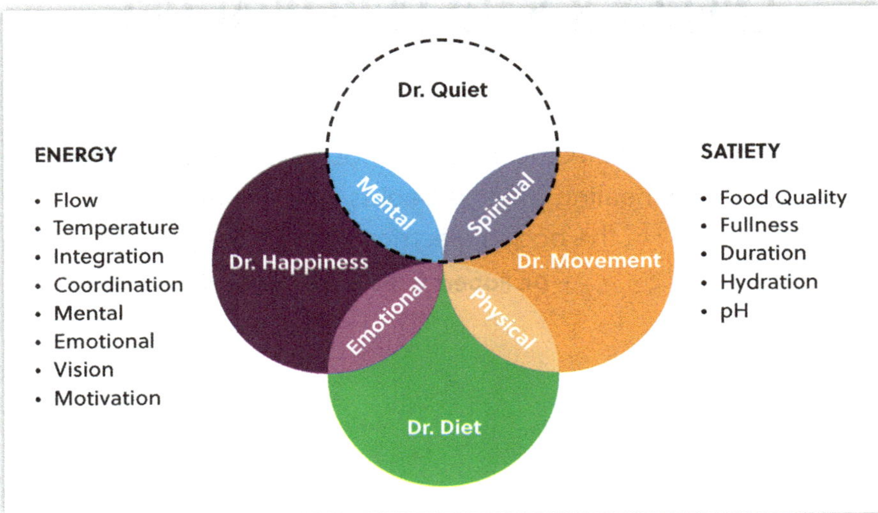

Figure 12: Diagram of Energy & Satiety

When these dimensions are balanced, we feel vital, creative, and free. When they are not, we are left tired, constrained, and pulled further away from health and purpose.

ENERGY: FLOW

Balanced energy flow sustains clarity, concentration, and emotional stability. When disrupted, it shows up as fatigue, depression, mania, or poor focus. Many people try to compensate with coffee, sugar, or energy drinks—stimulants that provide short-term relief but lead to cycles of dependency and burnout. Even professional athletes, who should model balance, often fall into this trap, as evidenced by the prevalence of energy drink sponsorships.

A healthy flow state arises naturally from whole food, restorative sleep, and living in sync with one's rhythms. Without this foundation, we swing between agitation and exhaustion, struggling to relax or sleep.

ENERGY: BODY TEMPERATURE

Body temperature is a window into health. Chronic inflammation elevates it, softening connective tissues and increasing risk of injury. Cold therapies—like ice baths—can be useful, but only when the body has enough reserves to adapt. People already stressed or fatigued often respond poorly, sometimes falling ill after cold exposure.

Patterns such as **night sweats** often point to underlying issues like parasite load or chronic inflammation, conditions far more common than most assume.

ENERGY: INTEGRATION

Integration is the body's ability to heal and adapt to life's stresses. When integration fails, we see burnout, inflammatory conditions, and tissue degeneration, such as osteoporosis, tendonitis, or spinal stenosis. I have seen athletes tear tendons so necrotic they had turned black. Such breakdown happens when nutrition, hydration, and rest are chronically neglected. Integration thrives when those foundations are honored.

ENERGY: COORDINATION

Coordination is more than athletic skill. It reflects harmony between nutrition, energy, and the nervous system. Stimulants like caffeine and sugar disrupt coordination, causing jitteriness, inaccuracy, and increased injury risk.

Simple balance tests reveal how diet shapes the nervous system. Athletes in precision sports, such as archery, martial arts or dance, know that breath control and clean nutrition restore fine coordination.

ENERGY: MENTAL

A balanced mind is coherent, creative, and adaptable. Imbalance leads to rigidity, impulsivity, forgetfulness, or chaos. Nutrition and lifestyle directly influence mental function: poor food and poor sleep erode clarity, focus, and emotional resilience. True mental health requires an integrated foundation.

ENERGY: EMOTIONAL

Healthy emotions naturally express empathy, compassion, and resilience. When out of balance, people fall into extremes—apathy (drained motivation) or fanaticism (rigid beliefs imposed on others). Both reflect weak dietary and lifestyle foundations.

Stress and poor nutrition lock the body into cortisol-driven patterns, making new habits feel threatening, even when change is desperately needed. This is why many resist eliminating foods that are clearly harming them.

ENERGY: VISION

Vision reflects both physiology and perception. Blood sugar imbalances blur vision, while poor visual tracking contributes to headaches, strain, and posture issues. Balanced vision supports orientation and focus. Imbalanced vision signals deeper systemic disharmony.

ENERGY: MOTIVATION

Motivation is the current that carries us forward. When well-nourished, we feel inspired to act and grow. When depleted, we cling to familiar but destructive habits. Poor diet keeps the body in survival mode, dampening motivation and reinforcing cycles of dysfunction.

SATIETY: FOOD QUALITY & FULLNESS

Satiety is more than "feeling full." It depends on food quality, digestive function, hydration, and variety. Poor-quality food leaves people hungry despite high calorie intake. Nutrient-dense food satisfies more deeply.

Hydration plays a central role. Many mistake thirst for hunger or cravings for soda, coffee, or juice. Processed, dehydrated foods demand extra water for digestion, weakening muscles and organs. Constipation, reflux, and bloating often follow, worsened by antacids and low stomach acid.

Addictions to gluten and dairy complicate satiety. Incomplete digestion of these proteins produces morphine-like compounds that soothe the brain, making withdrawal difficult. Combined with lack of variety—most people rotate between only 10-12 foods—this creates deep nutritional ruts.

Mindful eating restores balance. By engaging all five tastes—sweet, salty, sour, bitter, and umami—we awaken the body's innate feedback system. This not only supports satiety but also enriches emotional satisfaction and metabolic balance.

Fine-tuning your diet requires more than numbers. It demands attention to energy, satiety, and the interconnected factors that shape vitality. By listening to the body's feedback and honoring these principles, food becomes not just fuel, but a tool for balance, creativity, and sustainable health.

One of the simplest ways to understand diet's influence on the body is through experimentation. Try eating only one type of food for a day—such as sweet potatoes, yams, or naturally sweet fruits—and notice how your body responds. The point is not to adopt extreme diets, but to observe how food quality and variety affect satiety, energy, mood, and focus.

A powerful strategy is to **eat across nature's color spectrum.** Blueberries, bananas, squash, leafy greens, and red meat all provide unique nutrients and protective compounds. Restricting yourself to a narrow range of foods, even so-called "healthy" ones, can lead to subtle deficiencies that, over time, erode health.

Variety also matters in animal foods. A balanced diet should include seafood, poultry, ruminants (beef, lamb), and pork, rather than relying too heavily on one source like chicken or fish. The same principle applies to plant foods: above-ground vegetables, root vegetables, legumes, and fruits each offer distinct benefits.

Preparation methods also change foods nutritional profile. Frying, baking, steaming, broiling, stewing, fermenting, and eating foods raw each provide different advantages. Fermented foods, in particular, support digestion, immune health, and even bone strength.

SATIETY: DURATION

Satiety is not just about feeling full—it's about how long energy lasts after eating. Digestive issues such as rapid transit or constipation interfere with this process, often tied to blood sugar imbalances. These, in turn, affect mood, concentration, and energy.

A practical way to measure digestive transit is with the **red beet test.** Eat red beets and note the time until the pigment first appears in your stool—that's your transit time. When the last traces appear, that's your retention time. Ideally, transit should take **14–16 hours** and retention **56–72 hours.** Significant deviations may point to food intolerance, parasitic burden, or even emotional stress influencing digestion.

SATIETY: HYDRATION

Hydration is essential for digestion and overall vitality. Too little water concentrates toxins, slows elimination, and weakens energy. Too much water, especially during meals, dilutes stomach enzymes and disrupts digestion. The best practice is to hydrate **between meals,** ensuring fluids are absorbed before food arrives in the stomach.

Diets dominated by processed, dehydrated foods, such as bars, powders, and packaged snacks, force the body to pull water from tissues just to digest them. This weakens muscles and organs, leaving the body prone to fatigue and injury. Adequate hydration is not simply about thirst; it is a **prerequisite for muscle function, metabolism, and resilience.**

SATIETY: PH BALANCE

Of all the subtle regulators of health, **pH balance** may be the most overlooked. Excess acidity creates inflammation, drains energy, and fosters disease. Signs include shallow breathing, headaches, poor recovery, cravings, fatigue, and chronic aches. Acidic conditions also favor fungi and parasites, which thrive in low-oxygen environments.

While high sugar and heavy meat intake can drive acidity, excessive grain consumption can do the same, even in vegetarians. On the other hand, excessive alkalinity brings its own risks: tremors, nausea, dizziness, or muscle spasms. Balance is key.

Acidity robs vitality by stripping electrons from the body. Balanced alkalinity allows electrons to flow freely, supporting energy, resilience, and what ancient traditions call **life force.**

CHAPTER 8

PUTTING IT INTO PRACTICE

"Long-term consistency beats
short-term intensity."

~ Bruce Lee

One of the simplest yet most powerful tools for improving your health is diet and lifestyle logging. It requires no special equipment, no advanced training, and is available to anyone. While some people may struggle with techniques such as muscle testing or soul connection, logging provides a practical foundation. Over time, it can help those processes become easier and more natural.

You can keep your records using a smartphone, a day timer, or a paper notebook. The most important thing is to have enough space to capture the details of your day. Avoid calendars with tiny boxes—they rarely give you the room needed for meaningful entries.

When logging, focus on four key areas:

1. FOODS EATEN: WHAT AND WHEN

Be specific. Instead of writing "chicken and salad," record "two pieces of chicken and one bowl of salad." Precision matters because vague notes make it difficult to see patterns later.

The CHEK system uses simple serving size guidelines:

- **Flesh foods** (meat, fish, eggs)—the size of your hand, excluding the thumb.
- **Produce** (fruits, vegetables)—the amount you can hold in one hand.

Following these standards makes it easier to analyze your intake and balance the ratio of animal to plant foods. A useful rule of thumb: fat and protein sources usually come from organisms with eyes, while most carbohydrate sources come from organisms without eyes.

Also note the **time** you ate. This is critical for tracking symptoms. Without it, you may not be able to connect how food influences your body.

2. DRINKS—AND THEIR SOURCE

Record what you drink, how much, and when. If it's soda, how much? If it's water, where did it come from? Spring? Tap? Filtered? Bottled?

Water quality is especially important. Parasite infections and other health problems are often traced back to water. Knowing the source and type of water you drink provides essential context for understanding your health.

3. SYMPTOMS AND BODY SIGNALS

Track not only what you eat and drink but also how you feel afterward. Headaches, fatigue, mood changes, digestive shifts, or even subtle emotional states can provide valuable clues. Timing matters: if you had breakfast at 8:00 and felt a headache at 9:00, note it.

Worsening of existing issues is just as important. If a sore shoulder flares up after fried food, that's useful data. Pay attention, too, to bladder or bowel changes—these often reflect shifts in your nervous system and stress levels.

Don't limit yourself to physical signs. Emotional stress, mental fog, or even a sense of being "off" are worth recording.

4. SLEEP AND RECOVERY

Log your bedtime, wake-up time, and the quality of your sleep. Do you feel rested? Notice changes such as puffiness under the eyes, skin tone, or unusual breath. These details can highlight how diet and lifestyle choices are impacting your recovery.

Other Helpful Things to Track

- **Temperature fluctuations**—Waking up sweaty? Always hotter than others?
- **Sexual performance**—A sensitive indicator of vitality and hormonal health.
- **Cravings**—What foods or substances are you drawn to? Caffeine? Sugar? Chocolate?
- **Exercise**—Note the type, duration, and intensity. Different intensities stress the body in different ways.
- **Energy and mood rhythms**—Your organs and glands are wired to your muscles and joints. Unexpected pain or fatigue often signals deeper imbalances.

Your body communicates constantly through these signals. By paying attention, you can recognize both deficiencies and excesses before they become bigger problems.

WAYS TO RECONNECT WITH YOUR FOOD.

Beyond logging, there are powerful practices that deepen awareness of how food shapes health. If you are having trouble discerning the impact of specific foods on your well-being, here are some practical strategies to enhance your awareness and connection with food.

1. Participate in a Slaughter

Witnessing the taking of an animal's life, whether through farming, hunting, or butchering, creates a deep respect for meat. It reminds us that food is not abstract—it's life being transferred. Overconsumption of meat, especially through industrial farming, disrupts both ecosystems and personal health. Experiencing the sacrifice firsthand helps re-establish reverence and balance.

2. Garden Barefoot

Growing your own food fosters respect for plants and the intelligence of nature. Walking barefoot in the soil also helps discharge built-up electromagnetic stress from modern living, restoring your connection to the earth.

3. Prepare Your Own Food

Cooking at home reconnects you to the origins of your meals. Farmers' markets and local producers offer not only higher-quality food but also a deeper sense of trust and safety in what you're eating.

4. Eat With Your Hands

Before forks and knives, humans ate with their hands. This tactile experience slows the pace of eating and enhances awareness. For some, it even reduces overeating by bringing mindfulness back into meals.

5. Compost

Returning food waste to the earth closes the cycle of nourishment. Composting keeps us mindful of waste, supports soil life, and reconnects us with nature's regenerative rhythm.

6. Practice Fasting

Going without food for most of the day—or using only tea, diluted juices, or water—can reset the body and help you reconnect with hunger. Modern culture often encourages eating out of habit, not necessity. Fasting teaches patience, self-awareness, and gratitude for nourishment.

Diet and lifestyle logging is far more than data collection; it is a tool of self-awareness. Combined with mindful practices such as gardening, cooking, fasting, and composting, it builds a living connection between you, your food, and the earth. The more consistent you are, the clearer your body's messages become, guiding you toward health, balance, and vitality.

HOMEWORK

1. Keep a daily log of everything you eat and drink, noting any symptoms and the timing of their appearance, for at least 21 days.
2. Make a list of foods based on frequency and volume (e.g., bacon and eggs daily = frequent; muesli occasionally = infrequent).
3. Prioritize foods by how often and how much you consume. These will be tested against your body's responses in the program.
4. Track any symptoms over 24 hours, including digestive or urinary issues.
5. Examine not just your food, but also household and personal products (toothpaste, deodorant, body care). Many commercial, non-organic products contribute to toxic load. Consider guidance from a holistic health professional as you evaluate and make changes.

CHAPTER 9

MUSCLE TESTING & SOUL CONNECTION

"There is a voice that doesn't use words. Listen."

~ Rumi

Your body already carries the wisdom you need to guide choices about food, portion sizes, and even preparation methods. The challenge is not a lack of knowledge but learning to listen. Muscle testing offers one way of doing this. By engaging the subconscious mind, you access the vast storehouse of information held in your cells and nervous system. Researchers such as Bruce Lipton suggest that the subconscious processes millions of times more data than the conscious ego. Whether or not one accepts the exact figure, the truth remains: most of our intelligence lies beneath conscious awareness.

Yet, we are conditioned to make decisions from the ego alone—a small fraction of our real capacity. Beneath the surface, your cells already know how to heal, grow, and reproduce. When you fail to tap this deeper current of wisdom, you miss guidance that could help prevent illness and restore balance. With so many of today's health challenges rooted in unresolved body issues, the ability to hear what your body is saying is not a luxury but a necessity.

Ironically, despite the growing number of doctors, therapists, and fitness experts, chronic disease continues to rise. In this sense, pain itself becomes a teacher. Persistent discomfort is rarely random; it is a signal that something fundamental is being overlooked. If ignored or suppressed, it will simply resurface in another form, often more loudly. I encourage students and clients to welcome the ***PainTeacher*** as a messenger, pointing the way toward a deeper truth about themselves.

Real healing and growth require active participation. You cannot truly love or care for others if you neglect yourself. Self-care is the soil from which genuine love grows. To pretend otherwise is to live a kind of falsehood. Muscle testing and soul connection are practical ways to participate in your own well-being. Both are forms of dialogue with the body, and both assume that the body is an intelligent partner in the healing process. Through these practices you gain access to the innate knowledge of repair, recovery, and resilience that the body already holds.

Still, it is not unusual to encounter frustration at first. The ego often resists surrendering control. A controlling personality, for instance, may fear what the body might ask them to change, and as a result their testing produces unreliable results. Others may hesitate because of attachment to foods or substances they rely on, such as coffee, alcohol, sugar, or even protein powders. If they fear losing those comforts, the answers they receive may be clouded. Belief systems can interfere as well. Someone convinced that a particular supplement is the only key to muscle growth may unconsciously override the body's messages.

Social bonds add another layer of complexity. Many foods are woven into our connections with others, for example coffee breaks, shared drinks, birthday cakes, holiday cookies. These rituals foster belonging, but they can also make it difficult to listen honestly when the body signals intolerance. Fear of being judged or excluded often overrides the quiet inner voice.

The value of muscle testing and soul connection is that they reveal how often we live from the surface mind while ignoring deeper wisdom. By training yourself to listen, you begin to notice how much of your decision-making is driven by fear, habit, or social pressure. Consider that the nervous system processes billions of bits of information every second, yet the conscious mind selects only a handful, most of which are filtered through survival concerns. No wonder our perspective can be narrow and reactive.

Spiritual growth, then, means expanding trust in the deeper intelligence of the body and soul. It asks for courage—to listen without editing, and to act even when the answer challenges comfort or habit. It also means learning to quiet the inner critic, that ever-present negative voice of the ego, so that subtler messages can be heard.

If you struggle to get clear results from muscle testing, do not be discouraged. Continue to keep a detailed log of your food and lifestyle habits, and at the same time work on cleansing the body, calming the emotions, and clarifying the mind. Over time, the practice becomes more reliable.

With that foundation in place, I can now introduce two simple methods of self-testing—the duckbill and the finger loop. These are practical entry points for anyone ready to begin a direct dialogue with their own body.

THE DUCKBILL TEST

To begin, form a "duckbill" shape with the index and middle fingers of your right hand, leaving about an inch of space between them. With your left hand, use the index finger and thumb to gently press against the duckbill, as though trying to close it. At the same time, resist with your right hand to keep the shape open.

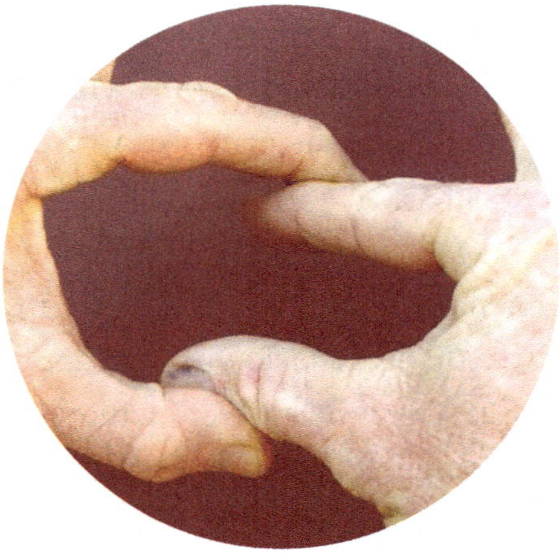

Figure 13: The Duckbill Test.

The goal at this stage is not to overpower the duckbill but to simply feel. Notice how much pressure it takes before the fingers begin to give way. This point, known in rehabilitation as the *breaking power* of the joint-and-muscle complex, is your reference baseline.

To understand why this matters, imagine performing a biceps curl. If your arm is bent and parallel to the ground, it takes considerable force from your other arm to push the working biceps down. Large muscles like the biceps have a high breaking force. For this reason, muscle testing is more effective when performed with smaller joints, where the subtleties of strength and weakness are easier to detect.

A common mistake is to apply too much force, trying to "win" against the duckbill rather than sense its subtle changes. The art lies in finesse, not brute strength. You are training yourself to feel the difference between strong and weak responses, not to overpower the muscle.

If you find the duckbill test awkward or difficult at first, don't be discouraged. There is a second option—the finger loop test—which some people find more comfortable and equally effective.

THE FINGER LOOP TEST

To perform the finger loop test, make a circle with the index finger and thumb of your right hand, as shown in Figure 14. Place the index finger and thumb of your left hand inside the loop, and then try to pull them through while your right hand resists. You will notice it takes a fair amount of force to break the loop. This baseline gives you a sense of your natural strength.

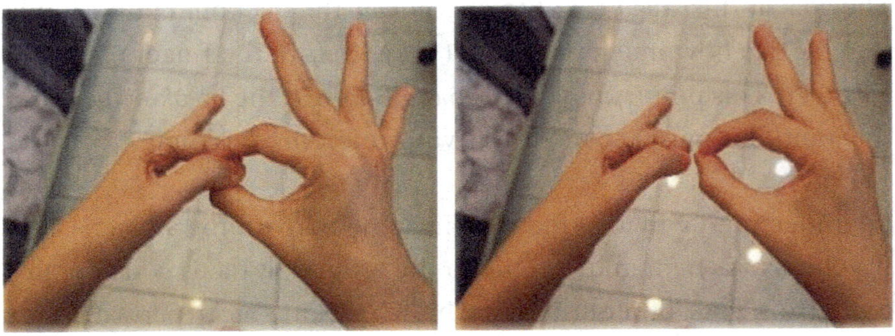

Figure 14: The Finger Loop Test

Some people find this test more comfortable than the duckbill, while others prefer the duckbill's sensitivity. Personally, I find the duckbill to be slightly more refined, but both methods are effective. The key is consistency—choose the one that works best for you but revisit the other from time to time to see which provides clearer results.

Once you've chosen your method, begin by asking your body a direct question. You can do this silently or out loud. For example, say: "Dear body, show me a yes through this muscle test." Resist firmly, holding the loop closed, and notice whether your effort feels the same as your baseline. Typically, your "yes" response will be about equal to your baseline strength. At the end of the test, I recommend saying "thank you," which signals that the communication is complete.

Next, ask: "Dear body, show me a no." In most cases, you will notice the loop weaken significantly. No matter how hard you try, you won't be able to keep it as strong as during the "yes" response. This contrast is the foundation of muscle testing: strength indicates yes, weakness indicates no.

Repeat once more by asking for a "yes," then test again, and say "thank you." Some people find that opening the duckbill or loop slightly wider makes the differences more obvious, but this is personal preference. Pay close attention to the variations—sometimes they are subtle, sometimes they are strikingly clear.

Over the years, I've worked with many clients who struggled to accept the validity of muscle testing. In those cases, I often offer a more definitive example. Imagine yourself as a primitive human, starving, when you stumble upon a large cluster of bananas. If you secretly kept them for yourself while your tribe went hungry, would this deception improve your chances of survival, or put you at greater risk? The answer is obvious: your survival depends on trust and cooperation. Similarly, your body's innate wisdom resists supporting self-deception.

This is why testing statements of truth and falsehood can be so powerful. Try saying: "Dear body, my name is [your actual name], and I am [your true age]." Then test. Most people remain strong. Now, give a false name or age, and test again. Almost without fail, the body weakens in response to the lie.

Skeptics may dismiss this as "airy-fairy," but history and science suggest otherwise. George Goodheart, an American chiropractor, and the founder of Applied Kinesiology in the 1960s, developed a systematic approach to muscle testing that has been widely studied and practiced. In his book *Applied Kinesiology: Synopsis*, Goodheart described how the body's physical responses are inseparable from emotional and mental processes. In other words, your body is always listening and always responding.

You can also begin testing foods. If you suspect you are not responding well to almonds, for example, place them in front of you, focus your attention on them, and test. The body recognizes not just the image of the food, but the full experience of eating, digesting, and assimilating it. This works for any food or drink—coffee, alcohol, desserts, or even your most common staples. In fact, the foods you eat most often are the ones most likely to reveal intolerances. While true allergies are usually genetic, intolerances often develop from repetitive exposure.

If you don't have a particular food on hand, simply visualizing it can still trigger a response. The subconscious recognizes the food image as clearly as the physical item.

USING THE TEST FOR THE 6 FOUNDATION PRINCIPLES

You can also apply muscle testing to the 6 Foundation Principles: breathing, thinking, movement, sleep, nutrition, and hydration. Simply ask:

- "Dear body, am I getting enough oxygen through breathing?"
- "Dear body, am I stressing myself with negative thinking?"
- "Dear body, am I getting the right amount of movement for health?" If the answer is no, ask whether you're doing too much or too little.
- "Dear body, am I getting enough sleep?"
- "Dear body, am I lacking specific nutrients in my diet?" If yes, you can review common nutrient lists to clarify further.
- "Dear body, am I well hydrated?" If not, consider not just volume but water quality, mineral content, and pH since much modern water is overly acidic.

The goal is to ask with clarity and intention so the answer can be expressed as a clear yes or no. Strong is yes. Weak is no.

Sometimes the body gives a "fuzzy" response, somewhere between yes and no. This is usually a sign that the question needs refinement. For example, instead of asking, "Should I eat more potatoes?" you might ask, "Should I eat one more serving of potatoes today?" A vague yes can often be sharpened by breaking the question into smaller steps.

FOOD PREPARATION, FLAVORS, AND COLORS

Your body may also guide you toward specific cooking methods, flavor profiles, or food colors. Each of these affects not only the taste of food but also its nutritional value. Open-flame cooking, for example, intensifies flavor but destroys delicate vitamins and minerals, whereas steaming or slow cooking preserves them.

Different flavors—bitter, sweet, salty, pungent, astringent, and sour—stimulate different receptors in the brain and regulate appetite. Modern diets often narrow down to just one or two flavor groups, leaving the appetite center unsatisfied. Asking which flavors your body needs can reveal nutritional gaps.

Food color is another way the body signals need. Each color corresponds to different nutrient classes: red, orange, yellow, green, blue, indigo, and violet all emphasize unique vitamins, minerals, and phytonutrients. If your body suggests a deficiency, you might ask, "Would more foods from the violet family help restore balance?"

Testing in this way encourages variety and balance across all food groups—seafood, poultry, ruminants, dairy, and plant foods—while also helping to identify potential problem foods. For example, pasteurized milk rarely tests positive, while pork often reveals intolerances.

PUTTING IT TOGETHER

These methods are not about rigid rules but about cultivating awareness. Muscle testing becomes a tool for self-education, teaching you to refine your diet and lifestyle according to your body's real needs rather than guesswork. Combined with the wisdom of the 4 Doctors—Dr. Diet, Dr. Movement, Dr. Quiet, and especially Dr. Happiness—this practice supports not only health but purpose.

When Dr. Happiness is clear—when you know your dream—choices around food, movement, and rest fall naturally into place. Without that clarity, we tend to use food as a drug, numbing frustration or loneliness instead of nourishing ourselves. Ultimately, the responsibility is ours. As adults, we must own our choices moment to moment.

Never forget that the subconscious mind is vastly more powerful than the conscious ego. When you ask your body whether to stay in a job, take more vacation, or make a change in diet, the answers matter. What stresses the mind stresses the body. What brings meaning to the mind brings meaning to the body as well.

SOUL CONNECTION

When I counsel people through relationship strain or conflicts with family and friends, I sometimes illustrate stress with a simple rubber band. I hold one end, invite them to pull the other, and ask them to match the amount of tension they feel around the situation; divorce, betrayal, loneliness, whatever is present. They usually pull hard. If either of us lets go, someone gets snapped. The point is straightforward: the farther we're pulled from our authentic center—away from presence and love—the more charge we build in the system. That charge must be resolved. The most efficient way forward is to listen for guidance from the quiet inner voice we call the soul, without coating it with our judgments or agendas.

Create the best conditions you can for that listening. Remove metal from the body, such as rings, earrings, nose studs, watches, fitness wearables etc, because they can act like antennas and add noise to a subtle conversation. Step away from televisions, radios, microwaves, and other sources of interference. Seek quiet. Soul connection asks for your full presence; if your space is noisy, move to one that isn't.

By "soul," I mean *consciousness within*. Huston Smith called it our "individual field of action." Rudolf Steiner described the soul's maturation in stages: a mineral level reflecting the body's basic elements; a biological or sentient level tied to the glands, organs, and the feeling life; an intellectual level where beliefs and identity form; and an awareness or spiritual level where honest self-reflection begins and received dogmas are tested. I offer this preamble only to clarify terms: we are speaking about the essence of our consciousness. When the body aches or feels off-center, it is a prompt to examine our choices—often starting with food—and to select what restores equilibrium.

Simple awareness drills can open this channel. Move your hand slowly toward your brow or the space between your eyes and notice the faint sensation, like the glow of a flashlight drawing near. Try the same with a phone: hold it at arm's length and gradually bring it toward your solar plexus, heart, or head; many people notice a change in buzz or pressure. Bring your hands toward each other as though collapsing an accordion. When they're an inch or two apart, most feel a subtle resistance, as if pressing into a cushion of air. These are small ways to sensitize yourself to fine energy.

A brief toning exercise helps, too. Sitting or standing, contract your left thigh for five seconds, then release and track where the energy travels. Do the same with the right thigh. Many feel a rising current toward the head. Now contract both gluteus muscles for five seconds, often the energy concentrates through the abdomen and solar plexus rather than the head. Continue with other groups—abdominals, lats, arms—and you've entered a progressive relaxation practice I first learned as a teenager with the Self-Realization Fellowship. Fifteen to twenty minutes of this prepares the system beautifully for meditation and soul work.

Next, shift your breathing. Place the tongue on the roof of the mouth just behind the front teeth. Inhale through the nose for a count of four, letting the belly expand first and the chest join only at the end. Hold gently for six. Exhale through the mouth for eight, keeping the tongue up and the abdomen relaxed; at the end, draw the navel inward to release stale air. Let a soft throat sound ride the exhale and imagine sending waste tension into the earth to be composted into something life-giving. Do four rounds. Practices like this decrease sympathetic tone, increase parasympathetic tone, and invite the right brain's broader, more integrative way of seeing.

Now you are ready to listen. Close your eyes and whisper, "Dear soul, if you can hear me, please show me what a *yes* feels like in my body." Breathe and feel. When you notice a response, say "Thank you." Ask, "Dear soul, please show me a *no*," and notice how it differs. Alternate yes and no a few times so your nervous system can map the contrast. One common question that follows is, "How do I know this isn't just my mind?" The answer is practice in receptive mode. Thinking has a felt texture—tightening, narrating, pushing. Listening is open, quiet, receiving. The essence of this work is deep listening that involves your whole being; as you enter it, the ego quiets naturally.

Bring this listening to everyday choices. If certain foods don't seem to love you back, ask inwardly while holding one food in mind at a time: "Dear soul, is this stressing me right now?" If the answer is yes, ask whether it should be removed for a period, and for how long. Many people need roughly three months away from a reactive food to let the immune system settle; confirm whether more or less time is appropriate. If removal isn't needed, ask about reducing frequency or portion—every other day, every third day, smaller servings.

You can do the same with the 6 Foundation Principles. Ask whether your breathing is effectively oxygenating you; whether you're thinking is creating stress; whether your movement dose is right or too much or too little; whether you are truly sleeping enough to recover; whether you are missing key nutrients; and whether you are adequately hydrated. If nutrition tests as a need, refine the dialogue: do you require more from the (choose one) red, orange, yellow, green, blue–indigo–violet spectrum; from above-ground vegetables, roots, fruits; or from particular food classes such as seafood, poultry and eggs, or ruminant meats? If hydration tests low, look beyond volume to water quality, mineral content, and pH.

Clarity hinges on how you frame the question. Yes/no queries work best. "Does my sister have brown hair?" is answerable; "What color is my sister's hair?" is not. If your signals feel fuzzy—a soft, mixed answer—tighten the question. Swap "Should I eat more potatoes?" for "Should I add half a serving of potatoes today?" Precision invites precision.

If the line still feels tangled, employ "soul clearing." See more about this in #4 below. The cleaner your inputs, the clearer your signal.

Remember that your soul is unconditional love—the very ground of consciousness. There is no shame in asking the same question more than once. Approach with humility and patience; you are in conversation with the most loving and trustworthy guide available to you.

Once you develop a profound sense of connection, gain awareness of your own soul, and possess the spiritual fortitude to confront the truth, begin to embark on a journey to explore deeper issues. Through years of practice and delving into the profound, I've witnessed firsthand the immense spiritual courage required to perceive God's intentions and, in this context, I use the term God not in the ethnocentric religious sense, but as a reference to the unified consciousness of all life and creation.

Soul communication is the pinnacle of spiritual practice, enabling direct access to the subconscious, superconscious, and universal consciousness. I highly recommend One Mind by Larry Dossey, a book that ranks among the top 20 books I have ever read.

THE TROUBLE SPOTS IN SOUL CONNECTING

There are several potential trouble spots that you need to recognize when it comes to tapping into your soul connection.

1. Soul communication is very subtle.

One who is internally or mentally preoccupied often loses the ability to sense soul communication. If you're overly stressed, you likely won't receive satisfactory responses from muscle testing. This is especially true when the ego's dominance overrides your feelings, causing it to feel the need to control everything and resist the realization that it can't have its way, whether it's a favorite snack or preferred beverage. Committing yourself to work-in practices like the zone exercises from *How to Eat, Move and Be Healthy!* and balancing yourself within the realm of your 6 Foundation Principles is often a prerequisite to effective soul communication.

In my experience, a person needs to dedicate themselves to a consistent 20 minutes daily of some form of tai chi, qigong, zone exercises, or breathing exercises, such as the 4-6-8 breathing method or other variations. Many of these practices are taught in various forms of yoga and in books on breathing or meditation.

Many people struggle to communicate with their inner selves due to their ego's fear of losing control, like muscle testing. If an individual lacks spiritual maturity to trust that there's a wiser and more complete entity beyond their intellect, they doubt themselves. Consequently, they block the communication between their subconscious, unconscious, and superconscious elements. These individuals often hold rigid beliefs and are driven by fear. They frequently encounter pain or the PainTeacher before they mature enough to realize their ability to guide themselves through life's challenges.

We learn that our individuality has limitations relative to the capacity that we have in relationship to others. It's crucial to be highly conscious, especially when seeking guidance from your soul on matters involving emotional connections, addictions, or personal desires, such as asking, "Was I fair to my wife last night during our argument?"

2. The ego learns to impersonate the soul.

It's common to encounter interference. Stress blurs perception. The ego dislikes losing control and will sometimes imitate the soul's voice, especially around charged topics like addictions or relationship conflicts. Before asking important questions, try a brief clearing: "Dear soul, please clear me of any disembodied energies or influences that could block our communication. Please give me a strong yes when we're clear." Many people feel an immediate quiet and a sense of clean space, as though static has lifted from the line.

I recommend developing your soul relationship with simple questions that don't challenge your ego or addictions, such as "What color shirt should I wear?", "What exercise would I like to do next?", or "How many minutes would I like to stay in the sauna today?" All of these are things that you don't really have an attachment to so that you can get your ego out of the way and become more aware of the presence of the energy and the feeling of how your soul communicates through you.

As sensitivity grows, you'll distinguish the soul's tone from the mind's push, and you can bring the practice into deeper matters. Over time, some receive images, some hear words, some experience a simple knowing. Each of us grows a personal language of the soul.

Your end goal is to develop that refined sense of when it is your soul talking or some other aspect of yourself, such as your ego, your fear, or anything else that you may have brought into your field, knowingly or unknowingly.

About that argument with your wife; if you're too childish and stubborn your ego may deceive you into believing you're right, causing more pain and problems in your relationship until you reach a breaking point and seek guidance from a counselor or even consider a divorce. Alternatively, you can grow up and realize that there's more to the situation than your ego can grasp and the best ways to learn are these types of practices.

3. Religious ideology is a common cause of inability to communicate.

Most often, this occurs with individuals raised in one of the approximately 30,000 branches of Christianity, where various forms of divination, such as dowsing (involving finding food and water in nature), are considered "the work of the devil." It's crucial to understand that the church employed these strategies to prevent individuals from developing self-sufficiency. Instead, they aimed to foster codependency on the church.

If you delve into Eastern religions, you'll see some experts refer to them as religions for adults because there's no central authority or deity providing guidance. In such systems, individuals are solely responsible for their actions and decisions, and connecting with their inner selves or the divine essence.

However, it is important to remember that any ideology that is worth living is worth challenging or testing. Connecting with your soul may invite you to look beyond inherited dogmas, not to diminish faith, but to deepen it into lived relationship. It may necessitate transcending religious dogma, but it can also provide a wide-open path to an abundance of creativity, love, connection, and a profound sense of support from the world, the universe, and the concept of God as understood by you.

4. You might be in the need of "soul clearing."

A crucial technique, especially since the ego enjoys impersonating the soul once it realizes it's losing control to something greater than itself, is to clear yourself. I'll share the technique momentarily, but I wanted to briefly explain how this happened.

I once had a case where I received a possession from a very sick woman in Toronto who had a lot of dark energy. Although this is the only time in my career that's ever happened, I was also feeling quite drained from traveling and speaking. After my lectures and working with her, I was walking to lunch when I felt an overwhelming sense of sadness and depression. This was very uncharacteristic of me, and I was trying to figure out what was causing it.

I was going to an organic cafe when the lady who owned it was in training with a spiritual master to become a healer. She was talking to me and seemed to be looking at me curiously. Then, she paused and said, "Paul, do you know that you have a possession? You have someone else's soul in your body right now." She asked if I was feeling okay. I admitted that I wasn't. She could sense that this soul was not a happy one, so she taught me a clearing technique right there and then.

This clearing technique effectively expelled that entity from me. Immediately afterward, it felt like someone had cleaned all my windows, and my energy surged, restoring my normalcy. That incident, in addition to the things I mentioned earlier, truly prompted me to realize that I needed to develop a technique for clearing. Through practice, I discovered all that I had to do was simply ask for what I desired.

Sit quietly and say, "Dear soul, please clear me of any disembodied souls, spirits, or entities that can block our communication. Please give me a strong yes when we're cleared." I encourage you to close your eyes and completely relax, paying close attention to your inner state. Those who struggle to distinguish between their ego and soul may discover a remarkable sensation: They can literally feel their soul moving objects around them, expelling energy. You'll also notice a profound sense of calmness within you, as if you were once talking on a poor phone connection then suddenly have perfect clarity.

Many of us carry various entities and spirits within us. For instance, alcohol is called "spirits" because it brings the spirit or consciousness of the plant into our bodies when we drink it. Smoking cannabis allows us to experience more of the consciousness of marijuana and how it lives. If consumed excessively, this can influence our thoughts, feelings, emotions, and decisions. Similarly, processed foods and meat can also affect our mental state.

5. Make eating a spiritual practice.

When consuming meat and vegetables, affirm to them that they are not dying but gaining life and love within you. Invite food and water into your being. It is spiritually important to recognize that when we consume food, if we kill an animal and eat it, its life is giving us life.

Furthermore, when we are conscious that we can carry the life of a plant or animal forward and use our life to support the life of nature, we become a living example for all human beings, inspiring them to have more love and respect for plants, animals, soil, water, earth, and sky. These are the elements that make up every one of us and we cannot live without them.

Therefore, eating becomes a spiritual practice of being aware that our lives are sustained by the sacrifices of other beings. Living this way opens our hearts and makes us more sensitive and capable of managing ourselves in ways that reflect loving intention rather than the typical Western "more is better" philosophy.

LONG-TERM SUCCESS

Fine-tuning diet is not about dogma or perfection. It's about **balance, variety, and listening to the body's feedback.** Long-term health requires meeting your body's needs—physical, emotional, and mental—day by day.

- Avoid rigid or overly narrow food choices.
- Let your body—not ideology—guide your nutritional decisions.
- Eat for **variety** across both plants and animals.

- Prioritize **quality foods**; cheap food often leads to expensive healthcare.
- Recognize the interconnection of **diet, movement, happiness, and sleep.**
- Consider a **four-day food rotation** to prevent nutrient gaps and intolerances.
- **Experiment with diet**: try eating only one type of food for a day (e.g., sweet potatoes, yams, or fruits) to observe how your body responds—energy, mood, satiety, and focus.
- **Avoid extremes**: the goal is not to adopt restrictive diets, but to learn how food quality and variety influence well-being.
- **Eat the color spectrum**: include a wide range of colorful foods (blueberries, bananas, squash, greens, red meat) to access diverse nutrients and protective compounds.
- **Balance animal foods**: mix seafood, poultry, beef/lamb, and pork instead of over-relying on one source like chicken or fish.
- **Balance plant foods**: include both above-ground vegetables, root vegetables, legumes, and fruits for full nutritional coverage.
- **Vary preparation methods**: cooking techniques (frying, baking, steaming, broiling, stewing, fermenting, raw) change food's nutrient profile.
- **Fermented foods**: especially beneficial for digestion, immune support, and bone health.
- Protect your **circadian rhythms** with adequate sleep.
- Honor your unique **Primal Pattern**® dietary needs.
- **Hydrate properly:** about half your body weight in ounces of high-quality water daily.
- **Limit processed foods and choose organic** whenever possible.
- Balance **resistance training and aerobic activity** to avoid deficiencies. Follow the principle: *work hard, rest hard.*

Walter Russell says the universe moves any idea or dream toward you at exactly the pace you move toward it. He says the universe operates on a 1:1 principle. For every step you make toward your dream, the universe brings your dream a step toward you. Every ounce of effort you put into it, the universe reciprocates, and my life experience has found that to be true.

REFERENCES

Brillat-Savarin, Jean Anthelme. *The Physiology of Taste.* 1825.

Chek, Paul. How to Eat, Move, and Be Healthy! CHEK Institute, 2004.

Williams, Roger. *Biochemical Individuality.* McGraw-Hill, 1998.

McCarrison, Robert. *The Cantor Lectures Delivered Before the Royal Society of Arts, 1936.* Royal Society of Arts, 1936.

Picton, L. J. *Thoughts on Feeding.* 1946.

Richardson, I. D. *Diet and Disease.* ME-NA Vita Co., 1932.

Cannon, Walter B. *Symptoms of Visceral Disease: A Study of the Vegetative Nervous System in Its Relationship to Clinical Medicine.* Literary Licensing, LLC, 2012.

Pottenger, Francis M., Jr. *Pottenger's Cats: A Study in Nutrition.* Pottenger's Nutritionals, 1983.

Price, Weston A. *Nutrition and Physical Degeneration.* Paul B. Hoeber, 1939.

Price, Weston A. *Nutrition and Physical Degeneration: A Comparison of Primitive and Modern Diets and Their Effects.* 6th ed., Price-Pottenger Nutrition Foundation, 2009.

CHEK. "The Organic Closed Cycle." *The Master Key*, 2024, myspiritgym.com.

CHEK. "The Wheel of Death." *The Master Key*, 2024, myspiritgym.com.

Worthington, Virginia. "Nutrition and Biodynamics: Evidence for the Nutritional Superiority of Organic Crops." *Biodynamics*, no. 224, July–Aug. 1999.

Goodheart, George J., Jr. *Applied Kinesiology: Synopsis.* 1964.

Dossey, Larry. *One Mind.* Hay House, 2013.

Made in the USA
Monee, IL
08 September 2026

62561394R00059